BASIC SKILLS FOR SURGICAL HOUSEMEN

BASIC SKILLS FOR SURGICAL HOUSEMEN

A GUIDE TO WARD PROCEDURES
FOR STUDENTS AND HOUSE OFFICERS

Kenneth C. Calman

LECTURER IN SURGERY, WESTERN INFIRMARY
GLASGOW

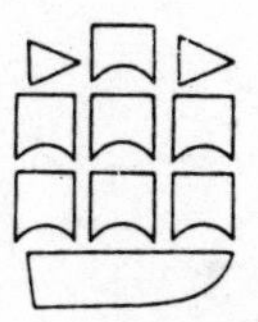

CHURCHILL LIVINGSTONE
EDINBURGH AND LONDON 1971

ISBN 0 443 00827 2

Filmset by Typesetting Services Ltd., Glasgow
and printed Offset by T. & A. Constable, Ltd., Edinburgh

PREFACE

There are many small books available to guide the medical student and house officer in the practical management of the patient in the surgical ward. Few, however, deal in detail with the techniques and procedures which the house officer will require to know for his day-to-day work in the wards. This small book attempts to bridge this gap by presenting, in a visual way, two aspects of the house officer's work. The first deals with procedures he will have to carry out on his own. The second deals with the preparation of patients for more complex and specialised procedures to be carried out by his more senior colleagues. These specialised procedures are described, to enable the house officer to appreciate the details of these techniques and thus more adequately prepare his patients. This book is not therefore a guide to management, but is a practical manual of ward techniques.

The responsibilities and duties of the surgical house officer vary widely from hospital to hospital. This simple fact makes it difficult to write a short book which meets the needs of all house officers, and a balance has to be achieved between what might be required in a major teaching hospital and what might be required in a peripheral hospital.

It must not, however, be assumed that this book will be sufficient in itself. There is no substitute for bedside demonstrations of a new technique. This is particularly the case with medical students working in the ward, who should not be expected to perform any of the techniques described without adequate initial supervision. In the first place it is unfair to subject the patient to inexpert or inexperienced hands. In the second place, should anything go wrong, there may be serious medico-legal consequences. This fact should be constantly borne in mind when duties are delegated to junior staff.

To avoid making the book too long, specialised neurosurgical, orthopaedic and paediatric procedures have been omitted, since several other books cover these adequately. Although this book has been written primarily for house surgeons, there may be some aspects of it which the ward sister or sister tutor may find useful for the explanation of procedures to her junior nurses.

This book could not have been completed without the advice and guidance of many colleagues in the Western Infirmary, Glasgow. I gratefully acknowledge their co-operation in reading the manuscript and their subsequent constructive criticism. To Mrs Jean Morocco of the Department of Medical Illustrations, the Western Infirmary, go my thanks for the beautiful illustrations of the techniques and procedures described in the text. I am also indebted to Miss Joanna Young who has deciphered and re-typed the many drafts of the book. Finally I should like to thank the staff of E. & S. Livingstone for their assistance in the production of this handbook.

1971 KENNETH CALMAN

CONTENTS

1. PREPARATION FOR OPERATION

In this chapter it will be assumed that after careful investigation and physical examination, a decision to operate has already been made. This section will therefore be devoted to the practical aspects of patient preparation prior to operation.

Explanation to the patient. As the patient is the focal point of any surgical procedure it is important that all relevant aspects of the operation are fully explained, preferably by the surgeon performing the operation. It is usual for the patient to be told the nature of his disease except perhaps in the case of malignancy. It is essential that the explanation given by the house surgeon is the same as that given to the patient by other members of the surgical team. Much of course will depend on the patient's illness and his reaction to it, but details of, and the reason for the operation should be explained in simple terms. It is helpful, for example, for the patient to know the site and size of the scar to expect, and whether a nasogastric tube, drain or intravenous fluids will be used post-operatively. The approximate time of the operation should be given to the patient. If a detailed explanation is given pre-operatively then much of the post-operative anxiety of patients will be allayed. With certain operations such as mastectomy, tracheostomy or abdomino-perineal resections a much more detailed explanation may be required.

Before the operation the patient must give his consent, in writing, to the anaesthetic and the surgical procedure to be performed. With gynaecological operations specific consent should be obtained before removal of the ovaries or uterus. Similarly, in males, if a testis is to be removed or the vas deferens divided because of disease, or prophylactically in the case of a hernia repair, prostatectomy or varicocele, consent should be obtained.

The details of the post-operative course should be outlined to the patient, and the importance of physiotherapy stressed. If possible pre-operative physiotherapy should be arranged particularly in the elderly and in patients with chronic lung disease.

Preparation of the patient for theatre. Before a surgical procedure, to be carried out under general anaesthesia, the patient should be fasted overnight. The operation site is shaved and the area washed with an antibacterial preparation. It is helpful to test the patient prior to operation for sensitivity to the skin preparation used, especially if the antiseptic contains iodine. Similarly allergy to adhesive tape may be tested for. The patient may require to be catheterised, have a nasogastric tube passed, or intravenous fluids commenced.

The technique of bowel preparation with a view to operations on the colon varies depending on the preference of the surgeon. There are essentially two aspects to the preparation: (1) the mechanical removal of faeces by enemas or suppositories, and (2) the use of antibacterial drugs. If three days are available for bowel preparation the patient should be placed on a low residue diet and given enemas daily together with phthalylsulphathiazole 2 g six-hourly. Alternatively neomycin (1 g six-hourly) may be given for 24 hours with repeated enemas until the lower bowel is cleared.

The most satisfactory method of bowel preparation requires five days and is as follows.

Day before operation	*Diet*	*Laxative*	*Enema*	*Antibiotic*
5	Normal	Liquid Paraffin	Suppositories	
4	Normal	Liquid Paraffin	Nil	Phthalyl-Sulphathi-
3	Normal	Liquid Paraffin	Enema	azole 4 g four times
2	Light	Liquid Paraffin	Nil	daily
1	Fluid	Nil	Enema b.d.	
0	Nil	Nil	Nil	

The theatre list. It is an important part of the house officer's duty to prepare, in conjunction with his senior colleagues, the order of patients for the operating theatre list. The ward nursing staff and theatre staff should be informed as soon as possible as to which patients will be going to theatre. In making up the operation list the full name, age and hospital number of the patient should be listed, together with disease and side of the body involved (i.e. left or right). It is a useful practice to mark the site of the operation on the patient prior to operation, in consultation with the surgeon performing the operation. This reduces the risk of operating on the wrong limb or wrong patient and facilitates identification in the operating theatre. If antibiotics or other drugs are to be given prior to the anaesthetic then they should be arranged at this time. Investigations to be carried out during the operation such as cholangiography, arteriography or immediate histological examination of a biopsy should be arranged with the appropriate hospital department.

Blood requirements for operation. Blood should be cross-matched prior to all but minor operations. It is difficult to give definite figures for each operation, and the surgeon performing the operation should be consulted. The following is a guide to requirements:

Mastectomy	1 litre
Thyroid operations	1 litre
Gastric operations	1–1·5 litres
Large bowel operations	1–1·5 litres
Vascular operations	2–3 litres
Amputations	1 litre
Thoracic operations	1–3 litres
Major cardiac operations	4–7 litres
Nephrectomy	1 litre
Prostatectomy	1 litre

Blood should be stored at 4 to 6°C, and should be removed from the refrigerator immediately before use. Blood should not be left at room temperature for any length of time before use.

Pre-medication. This should be arranged in consultation

with the anaesthetist. For most operations in adults under general anaesthesia, atropine (0.6 mg) or scopolamine (0.4 mg) is given intramuscularly 30–60 minutes prior to the anaesthetic. A sedative drug, usually morphine (10–15 mg) or papaveretum (Omnopon) 15–20 mg) is given at the same time. For procedures under local anaesthesia or for endoscopic examinations the drugs detailed above may also be given; alternatively sedation by intramuscular or slow intravenous injections of diazepam (Valium) (5–10 mg) may be used to induce both sleep and detachment of the patient.

Explanation to the relatives. This is an important part of patient care in which the house officer is often involved. For most patients, and certainly for those undergoing major operations, the patient's relatives should be informed of the operation, the disease and possible complications. This should be done before operation. Relatives are often worried about post-operative drips and tubes and these fears can be allayed by pre-operative explanation. Such explanations are usually given by the surgeon performing the operation but the house officer may be asked either to confirm or amplify them. In difficult situations it is therefore important that the advice of a senior colleague is obtained before speaking to patient's relatives.

2. LOCAL ANAESTHESIA

Many different local anaesthetic preparations are available but agents such as lignocaine, procaine or other similar proprietary preparations in concentrations of 0.5 to 2 per cent, with and without adrenaline are most useful. The addition of adrenaline acts as a vasoconstricting agent, diminishes bleeding and increases the duration of action of the local anaesthetic. Adrenaline in a local anaesthetic solution must never be used in the fingers or toes, in the ears or in the penis, since this may result in vascular spasm with subsequent gangrene of the part. Nor should adrenaline be used in inflamed tissue or the traumatised urethra. For most purposes a 1 per cent solution of lignocaine is all that is required. Adrenaline at concentrations of 1 in 200,000 is adequate. The maximum dosage of local anaesthetic which should be given in the adult is 200 mg without adrenaline (20 ml of 1 per cent solution) and 500 mg if adrenaline is used (50 ml of 1 per cent solution). These doses should be reduced in the elderly patient.

As with all surgical procedures an adequate explanation of the procedure must be given to the patient. There will of course be pain as the needle is inserted through the skin and, as the local anaesthetic is infiltrated, there is often a momentary stinging sensation which soon disappears. Remember that although sensation will be abolished in the area which has been infiltrated, the patient will still retain normal sensation outwith this region. Pressure may still be experienced and the patient should be warned that not all sensation will be lost. It should also be noted that carelessly placed instruments or towel clips will soon be noticed by the patient. Following the use of local anaesthesia transitory paralysis may result; this should be explained to the patient, particularly if the region to be anaesthetised involves the face.

Local infiltration of the skin and underlying structures (Figure 1)

After cleansing the skin with antiseptic solution a bleb of local anaesthetic is raised intradermally using a fine needle (23 gauge). This is allowed to act for a few seconds then the needle is inserted more deeply. Care should be taken not to enter any of the blood vessels in the dermis or subcutaneous tissue and should be checked by gentle withdrawal of the plunger. If more extensive or deeper infiltration is required a longer needle with a wider bore (18–20 gauge) should be used. This technique allows the infiltration of local anaesthetic to a limited area and is suitable for procedures in which needles or drains are to be inserted.

For the removal of lesions within the skin the local anaesthetic is injected around the lesion through one or more sites. For wound suture the local anaesthetic is injected into the skin through the edges of the wound. The needle is inserted for its full length along the line of the wound, the plunger is withdrawn to check that the needle is not in the blood vessel and local anaesthetic is injected. The needle and syringe are then withdrawn a little and the manoeuvre repeated until the whole length of the wound is anaesthetised.

Anaesthesia of the fingers and toes (Figure 1)

This may be conveniently carried out by infiltration of the local anaesthetic (1 per cent without adrenaline) on either side of the finger or the toe. The needle is inserted into the dorsal aspect of the skin web and directed towards bone where the digital nerves lie. This process is repeated on each side of the finger, 0.5 ml being injected at each site. Alternatively the 'one prick technique' may be used. A bleb of local anaesthetic is raised over the dorsal aspect of the finger or toe and through this anaesthetised area both sides of the digit are anaesthetised. If the local anaesthetic has been placed in the correct site, the finger will soon become anaesthetised. For control of bleeding a rubber tourniquet is placed around the finger by rolling it on from the fingertip. This must be removed at the end of the procedure and a note of the tourniquet time made.

INFILTRATION OF LOCAL ANAESTHETIC SOLUTIONS

SKIN-LEVEL OF INFILTRATION

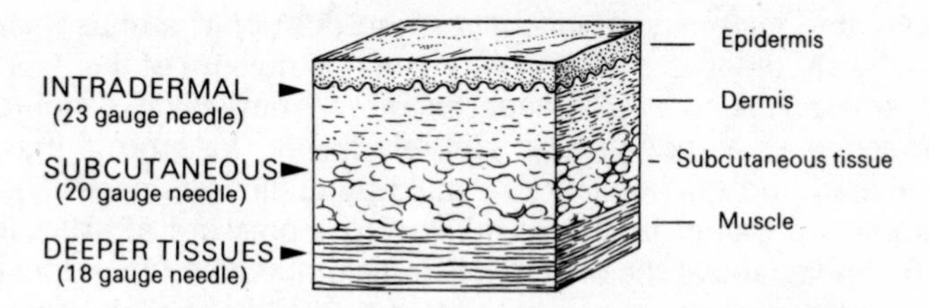

LOCAL ANAESTHESIA FOR A SMALL LESION

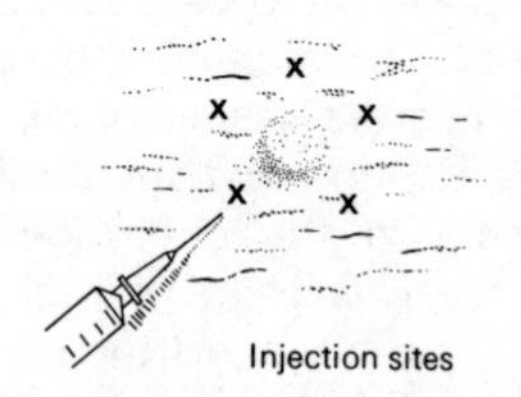

LOCAL ANAESTHESIA OF AN OPEN WOUND

Needle inserted then withdrawn as anaesthetic injected

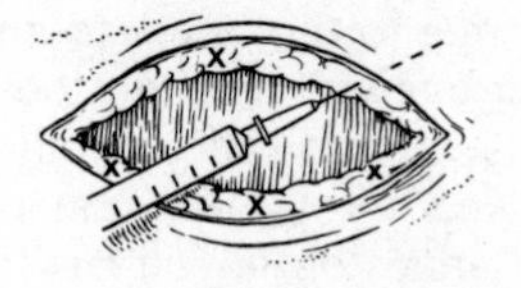

ANAESTHESIA FOR FINGERS AND TOES

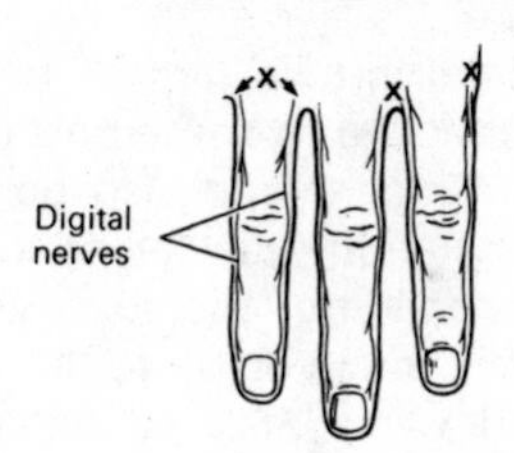

Figure 1

Anaesthesia of the upper limb (Figure 2)

Anaesthesia of the upper limb may be readily accomplished by intravenous administration of local anaesthetic agents. This technique is suitable for such procedures as reduction of fractures of the limb.

Two tourniquets are necessary, usually in the form of sphygmomanometer cuffs, placed on the upper arm as near to the shoulder as possible. A vein on the dorsum of the hand is entered using a 20 gauge needle or indwelling cannula attached to a syringe, and securely fixed. The limb is then elevated and the veins are emptied by gravity drainage. The upper tourniquet is rapidly inflated to a pressure of at least 50 mm Hg above the patient's systolic blood pressure. A local anaesthetic solution (0.5 per cent without adrenaline) is then injected at a dose of 3 mg/kg of body weight, usually 30 to 40 ml in the adult. The needle is then removed and firm pressure applied to the venepuncture site for at least five minutes. When anaesthesia is complete the lower tourniquet is inflated and the upper one released. This manoeuvre avoids pain due to the upper tourniquet since the tissues under the lower one will be anaesthetised. This tourniquet should then be securely fixed and the pressure in the cuff regularly checked throughout the procedure. This form of regional local anaesthesia will last for up to two hours. At the end of the procedure, or after a minimum of at least 20 minutes, the tourniquet is released gradually over a period of five minutes to prevent flooding the systemic circulation with the local anaesthetic agent.

Intercostal nerve block

This procedure is useful in relieving the pain of fractured or bruised ribs. To be effective two intercostal nerves above and below the fractured ribs should also be anaesthetised. The needle is inserted posteriorly, just lateral to the transverse process of the corresponding thoracic vertebra. Local anaesthetic solution is infiltrated down to the level of the rib. The needle is then withdrawn a little, redirected, and inserted at a slightly lower level so that it is located at the inferior border of the rib where the intercostal nerves lie. Aspiration

REGIONAL INTRAVENOUS ANAESTHESIA

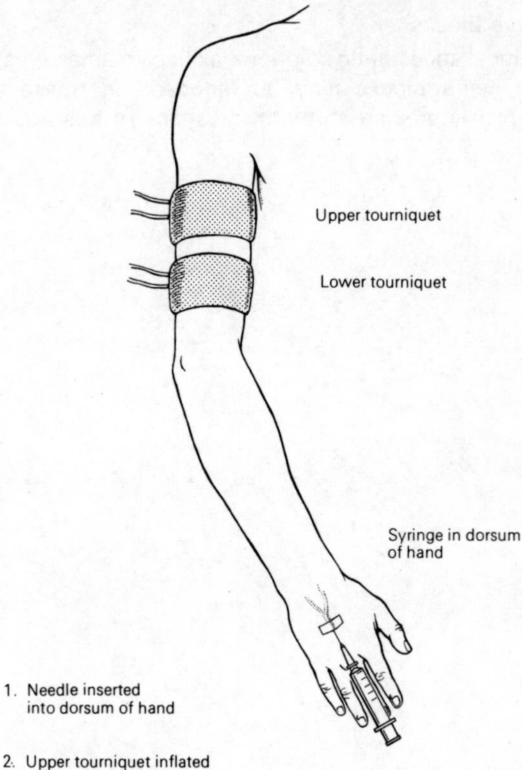

1. Needle inserted into dorsum of hand
2. Upper tourniquet inflated
3. Needle removed and firm pressure applied
4. When anaesthetic effective lower tourniquet inflated and upper one released

Figure 2

of the syringe should be performed to check that the needle is not in a blood vessel before 2 ml of 1 per cent local anaesthetic (1 per cent without adrenaline) is injected.

Local nerve blocks

Using local anaesthetic solutions, axillary, palmar, wrist and pudendal nerve blocks may be induced, but these more complex procedures are outwith the scope of this book.

3. THE CARE OF WOUNDS

Introduction

A great deal of the house surgeon's work is concerned with the care of wounds; the insertion of stitches, the removal of stitches, wound infections and wound dehiscences. Most important of all however, at least to the patient, is the problem of wound pain. Many of the procedures to be described here may be carried out by the nursing staff, but it is important that the house surgeon is familiar with the techniques involved.

Cleaning and debridement of wounds (Figure 3)

Cleaning and debridement of traumatic wounds are mandatory prior to closure. Local anaesthesia is performed as described in Chapter 2. Cleaning is accomplished by washing the wound edges and deeper structures with saline or a mild antiseptic solution such as aqueous chlorhexidine (0.1 per cent). All foreign bodies and dirt should be removed by scrubbing if necessary. Having cleaned the wound, the edges and deeper structures are examined carefully. Except in the case of clean incisions the wound edges should be trimmed. Areas suspected of being non-viable, by virtue of a bluish colour and diminished capillary return on pressure, should be excised until bleeding occurs, along with damaged muscle. Failure to remove such necrotic tissue may lead to poor wound healing or even to gas gangrene. As a prophylactic measure patients with traumatic wounds should be given the first injection of a course of tetanus toxoid together with a long-acting penicillin.

The closure of wounds (Figure 3)

This is a skill which can be obtained only by practice under supervision, but the following points may be useful.

Needles to be used. Atraumatic needles, that is needles with an attached stitch, are generally preferred. For skin sutures, 3/0 (000, 2 Metric) black silk or linen is used. For

WOUND CARE I

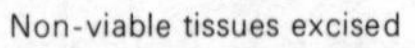
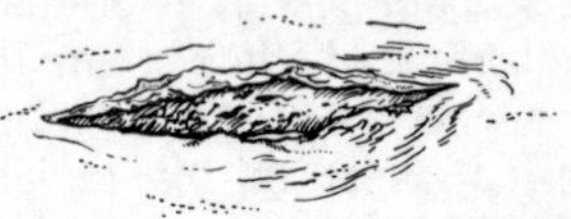

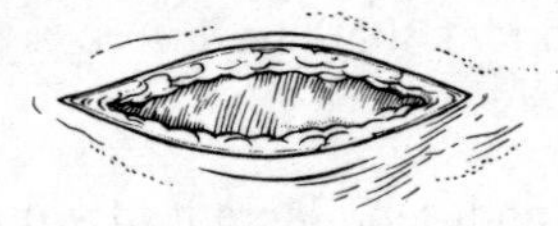

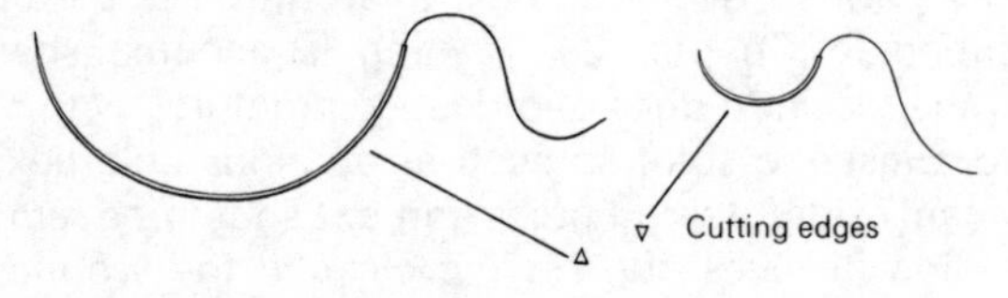

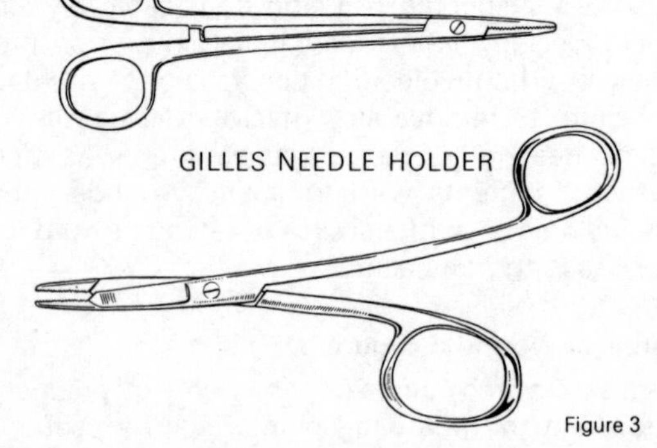

Figure 3

facial wounds, a finer material, usually 5/0 (1 Metric) silk, is preferred. Some needles are large enough to be used by hand but the smaller ones will require a needle holder.

Needle holders. Various types of needle holders are available; most have jaws held by a spring clip. One type of needle holder, the Gillies, does not have a spring clip but it does have scissors incorporated into the blades.

Insertion of stitches (Figure 4). For most wounds the stitches should be inserted approximately 0.5 to 1 cm apart. Equal bites of the skin should be taken so that the edges lie correctly together and the stitches tied as shown. For most facial wounds smaller bites should be taken and stitches inserted at more frequent intervals.

Closure of wounds by adhesive tapes (Figure 5). This method of wound closure is convenient in some cases but certain precautions should be taken before use. The skin and wound should be thoroughly cleaned as described above and all bleeding within the wound should be stopped before the tapes are applied. If the wound is superficial then the tapes may be applied directly. If, however, the wound is deep or there is excess fat, then subcutaneous stitches of an absorbable material such as 3/0 (2.5 Metric) plain catgut should be inserted first. When the wound is completely dry the tapes are applied without tension on the wound, otherwise friction blisters may occur.

Post-operative wound care

Control of wound pain. To the post-operative patient this is a most important aspect of his operation. Post-operative wound pain is usually present for the first few days after operation. At first it is constant but eventually is present only on moving or coughing. If continuous wound pain persists longer than this then it is likely that there is some pathological process, such as a wound infection present. In the first 24 hours post-operatively wound pain can usually be controlled by morphine or omnopon given subcutaneously every four to six hours. The dosage and drug used will depend on the weight and the age of the patient. For a small person 10 mg

WOUND CARE II

INSERTION OF STITCHES

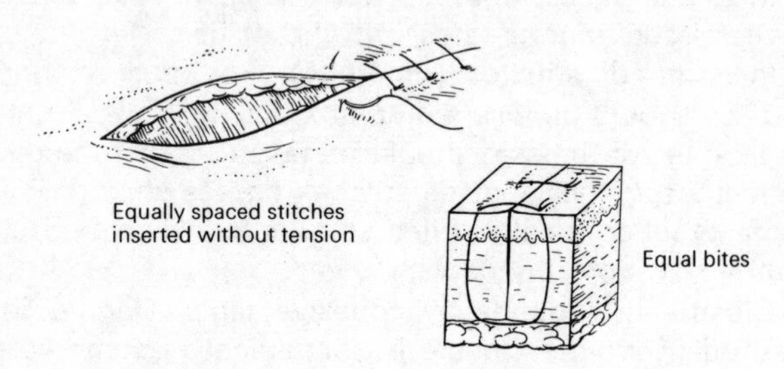

METHOD OF INSERTION OF STITCHES

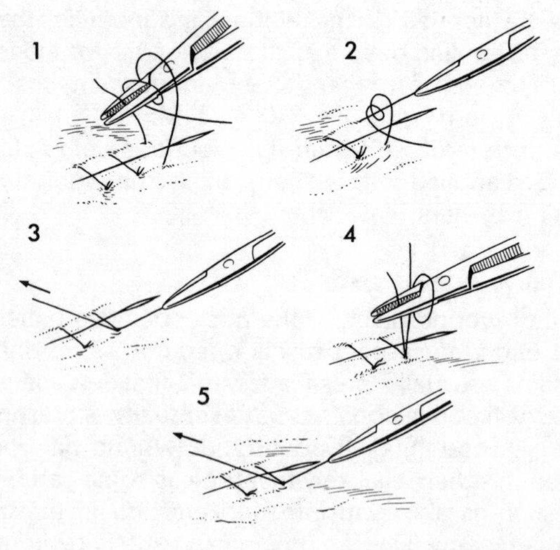

Figure 4

of morphine will be sufficient. For the heavier person 15 mg of morphine or 20 mg of omnopon may be used. In the elderly patient the effect of these drugs is often more pronounced and they should be used with great care. It should not be forgotten that these drugs can cause respiratory depression and this must always be borne in mind.

In some cases it is more convenient to give these drugs intravenously, and in smaller doses given at more frequent intervals. In this way the dose of analgesic may be titrated to the level of the pain. With this technique, 10 mg of morphine are diluted with 10 ml of sterile saline and 1 to 2 ml of this solution given three hourly, or more often if required. After the first 24 hours, the dosage and frequency of these drugs may be reduced and the patient given either 30 to 60 mg of pentazocine hydrochloride or 50 to 100 mg of pethidine by intramuscular injection every four to six hours. This routine however may not apply to all cases; thus the phantom limb pain which may follow amputation often continues for some time, and requires considerable quantities of analgesics. The danger of addiction to these drugs with prolonged use must be constantly borne in mind and they should be stopped as soon as possible.

Wound infection

The aetiology of wound infections in general is not considered here. Suffice it to say, that post-operative wound infections still remain a cause of considerable morbidity. In most cases the diagnosis is obvious. The patient's temperature is elevated, the wound is inflamed, swollen and tender, and there may be a discharge of pus. In such cases the principle of drainage of the wound should be observed and if necessary one or more stitches should be removed from the most inflamed area, sinus forceps inserted and gently opened to allow free drainage of pus. If the pus is draining there is usually no need to give antibiotics as the infection will settle within a few days. A swab should be taken however to identify the organism and test sensitivity to antibiotics.

WOUND CARE III

REMOVAL OF STITCHES

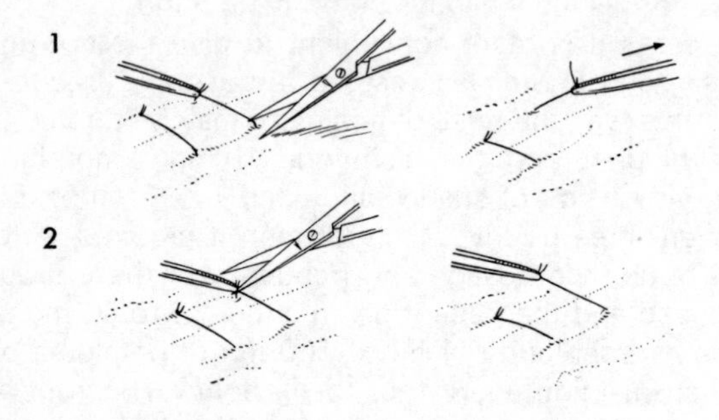

TAPE CLOSURE OF WOUNDS

Tapes equally placed without tension
Interrupted catgut inserted if wound deep

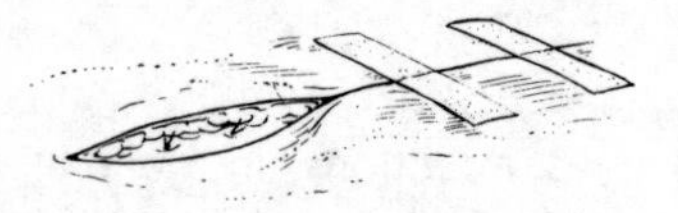

Tapes evenly applied
Edges held by forceps

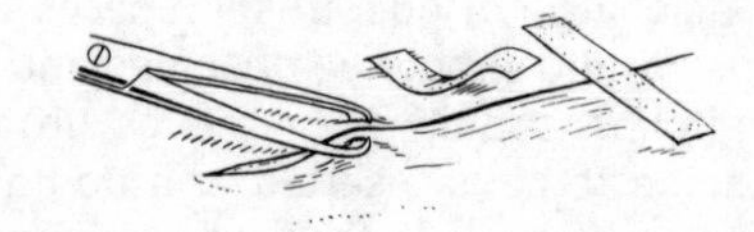

Figure 5

Wound dehiscences

In a small proportion of post-operative patients the wound ruptures exposing the underlying structures. If the dehiscence is superficial, that is the skin only is involved and the deeper layers are left intact, the opening should be packed with a suitable antiseptic dressing such as chlorhexidine, and daily dressings of the area carried out until the wound is clean. At this stage it may be left to granulate or may be closed as a secondary procedure.

If all layers of the wound are involved, a different picture is seen. For a few days prior to rupture there is often a sero-sanguinous discharge. The dehiscence may appear to be superficial at first, the deeper layers remaining intact. Gradually however, over a period of hours the dehiscence becomes complete and, if it is an abdominal wound, coils of bowel or omentum can usually be seen. When this occurs the diagnosis of complete rupture can be made with certainty. The wound should be covered with warm saline-soaked swabs or packs. In the case of abdominal or thoracic wound rupture the patient should be prepared for theatre and immediate re-suture performed.

Removal of stitches and tapes (Figure 5)

It is surprising how many patients are apprehensive about this simple procedure. Once again, reassurance by the doctor may help to relieve this fear. To remove stitches, the wound and surrounding skin is first cleaned with antiseptic solution such as aqueous chlorhexidine. Using sterile forceps and scissors, or a stitch cutter, the suture is first elevated by the forceps and the stitch cut as close to the skin as possible, then removed. Cutting the stitch in this way avoids pulling contaminated suture material through the wound. After removal the area is again cleaned with an antiseptic solution.

With tape closed wounds, the tapes are left in place for 7 to 10 days and then gently removed by traction. This technique should be explained to the patient as he can usually remove his own tapes after discharge from hospital.

4. VENOUS BLOOD SAMPLING

Equipment required. Before approaching the patient have everything at hand. Syringe, needle, swabs, venous tourniquet and specimen tubes ready labelled. In the interests of efficiency a small tray containing these items makes it easier to deal with several patients.

Preparing yourself and the skin. The hands should be washed before taking blood but a mask is not necessary. After selecting a suitable vein, the area should be prepared by washing with an antiseptic solution such as 5 per cent chlorhexidine in 70 per cent alcohol.

Approaching the patient. Remember that the patient in hospital is often anxious and worried about his illness. Reassure him and explain to him in detail what you intend to do, and tell him the reason for the venepuncture so that he can co-operate more fully. If possible keep the needle and syringe out of sight until the last moment.

Sites for venepuncture (Figure 6)

The ante-cubital fossa. This is the most commonly used site; the veins are usually large and easily visualised. Although the pattern of veins is not constant a typical arrangement is shown in Figure 6.

Forearm veins. Venepuncture, though easy in these sites, tends to be painful. The cephalic vein at the level of the radial styloid is often large and convenient for venepuncture.

Veins of the dorsum of the hand. Once again venepuncture at this site is often painful.

Femoral vein. This vein should be used as a last resort. To locate this vein, first palpate the femoral artery in the groin. The artery is situated midway between the anterior superior iliac spine and the symphysis pubis. The femoral vein is just medial to the artery (for details see section on Femoral Vein Stab, pages 24–25).

Application of the venous tourniquet. This should be done as gently as possible, proximal to the site of the venepuncture.

SITES FOR VENEPUNCTURE

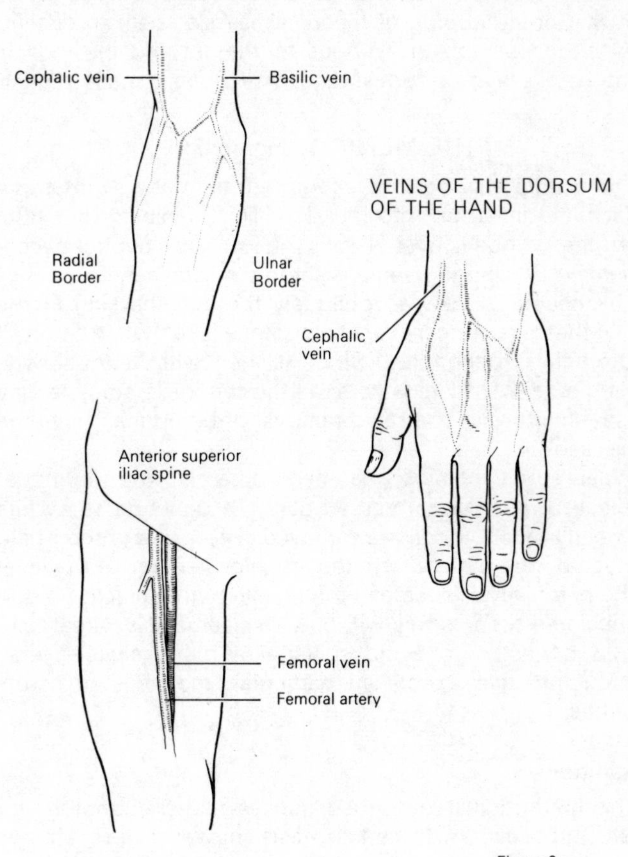

Figure 6

A co-operative patient may be able to occlude his own veins using his other arm. If not, then a rubber tube, proprietary tourniquet, or sphygmomanometer cuff may be used. In most patients, veins distend quickly using the tourniquet alone. If the veins do not fill quickly, ask the patient to open and close his hand. This increases the venous return because of increased muscular activity and the veins distend more rapidly. Gentle tapping of the vein may also help to distend it. Although useful, the venous tourniquet and the muscle pump have several disadvantages which are discussed later.

THE METHOD (Figure 7)

The needle may be used straight, or bent at a slight angle to facilitate insertion into the skin. This is especially useful when the syringe is over 20 ml in size or has a central needle fitment. A 20 gauge needle is the most satisfactory.

The needle is inserted obliquely through the skin in the line of the vein. A decrease in resistance is felt when the wall of the vein is penetrated. Blood is then withdrawn slowly, making sure that there is no air in the syringe, since this may cause haemolysis. Too rapid removal of blood may have the same result.

When sufficient blood has been obtained, the tourniquet is released. A swab is pressed over the puncture site while the needle and syringe are removed. The swab is then held in place by the patient with the arm elevated above the level of the heart. Always remove the needle before placing blood in specimen tube as this will prevent haemolysis. Great care should be taken to avoid spillage of blood since it may contain infective agents, in particular, the virus of serum hepatitis.

Precautions

The method just described applies to venepuncture for most purposes. With certain tests however, precautions must be taken.

Use of the tourniquet. It is important, of course, to make sure that the tourniquet is not too tight or the arterial supply

METHOD OF VENEPUNCTURE

1. Needle inserted obliquely into the skin

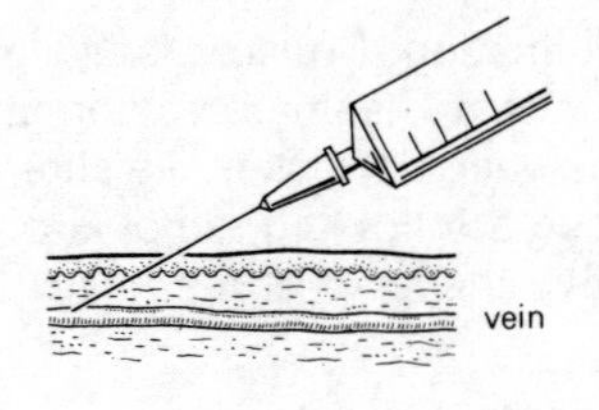

2. Needle inserted in line of vein

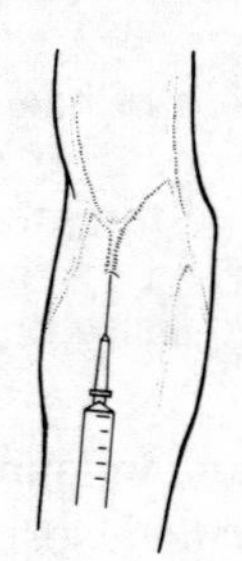

3. Blood gently withdrawn then needle removed

4. Elevate arm above level of the heart

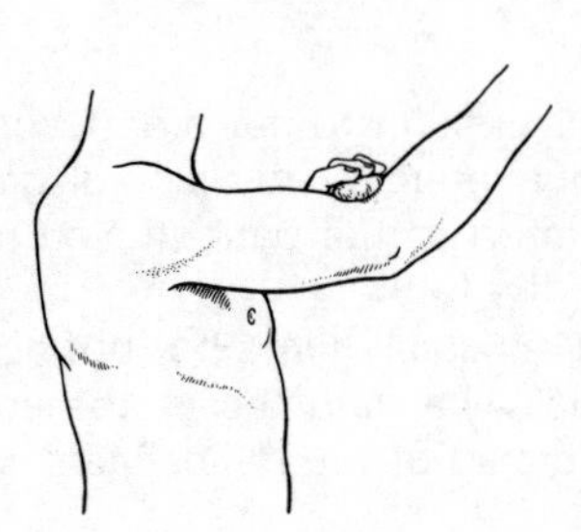

5. Remove needle and dispose of it carefully
Fill specimen tubes

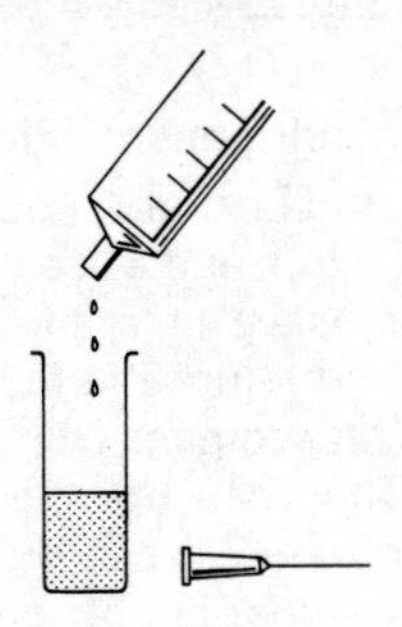

Figure 7

will be reduced and the venous return decreased. Blood samples for platelet counts and blood calcium estimation require that the tourniquet should be loosened after insertion of the needle and before taking blood.

Using the muscle pump. This is a very useful technique to aid distension of veins but has its disadvantages. The serum potassium for example, can be significantly raised by this procedure and it should not be used unless absolutely necessary.

Prevention of haematoma formation. Bruising is unsightly to the patient, and more important, haematoma formation may result in thrombosis of the vein. Always make sure that haemostasis is adequately secured following removal of the needle, by raising the arm above the level of the heart.

Venepuncture in jaundiced patients

In any patient suspected of having infectious hepatitis, or in any patient with jaundice of unknown aetiology special precautions should be taken. Gloves should be worn and great care should be taken to avoid spilling blood. Specimens should be sealed and placed in polythene packets and sent to the laboratory. The laboratory should be consulted fully before such specimens are sent, and the specimen forms should be labelled accordingly.

The difficult patient (Figure 8)

Remember that if you find it difficult to get blood from a patient, stop, and ask a colleague for help. This is no disgrace and may save time and discomfort to the patient. You may be able to return the favour in the future.

The fat woman. The veins are usually large but not easily seen. They can however, usually be palpated in the antecubital fossa or seen on the dorsum of the hand. Make sure the tourniquet is not too tight.

The thin old patient. The veins are sclerotic and jump away from the approaching needle. It is a mistake to try to spear the vein. Rather, the needle should be inserted about 1 cm distal to the proposed point of insertion, and the vein held by

THE DIFFICULT PATIENT

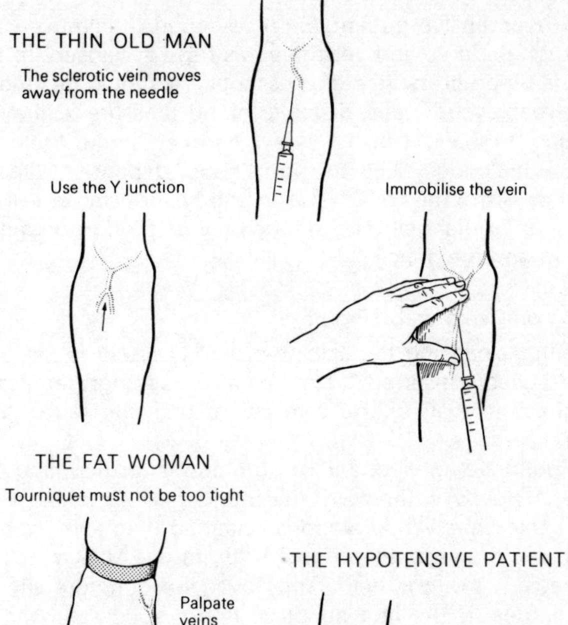

Palpate veins

Use dorsum of hand

THE HYPOTENSIVE PATIENT

Use sphygmomanometer

Figure 8

traction of the skin with the fingers of the left hand prior to being entered. If possible a Y junction in the vein should be looked for since this is often a very useful site for venepuncture.

The hypotensive patient. Blood is often required quickly from such patients and yet the veins have collapsed. In this case the blood pressure cuff is essential. It should be inflated to between systolic and diastolic blood pressure. It may be necessary to leave it on for a few minutes before the veins become distended. Let the arm hang dependent and if necessary warm the limb. If this method is not successful the femoral or jugular vein may be the only method of obtaining blood in an emergency.

The femoral vein stab (Figure 9)

1. After cleansing the skin the femoral artery is palpated and the needle inserted 1 cm medial to it at right angles to the skin. The wall of the vein can usually be felt as it is pierced.

2. Suction is applied, and, if no blood is forthcoming, the needle is slowly withdrawn, the plunger being pulled back at the same time. When blood is obtained the needle is held steady and the required amount withdrawn. After removing the needle a swab is held firmly over the puncture site for two minutes. If the first puncture is not successful then a second site should be tried. Remember that the femoral vein is usually deeper and more medial than expected.

BLOOD CULTURES (Figure 10)

The doctor must thoroughly wash his hands, scrub his nails and wear a mask. The hands are dried on a sterile towel and gloves are worn. The tourniquet is applied by an assistant. The patient's skin is prepared by washing with antiseptic solution then dried with a sterile swab held with sterile forceps. It is important that excess antiseptic is removed in case it is transferred to the culture bottles.

Without touching the skin with the right hand the needle

THE FEMORAL VEIN STAB

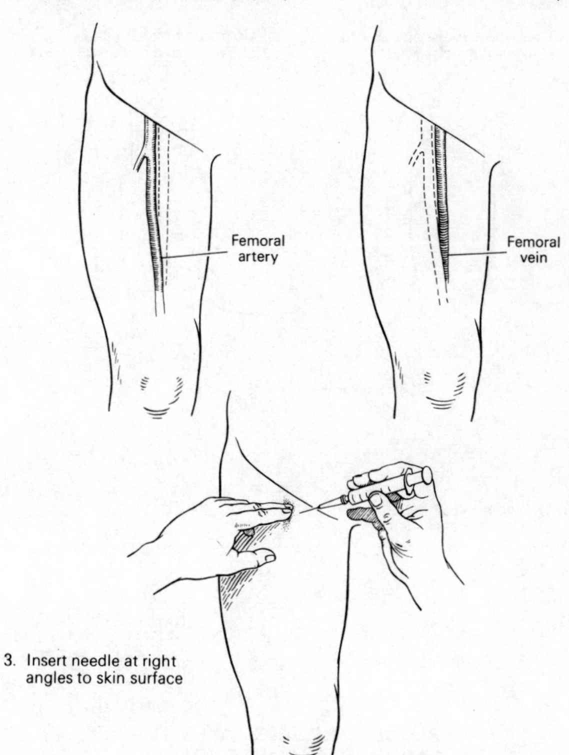

Figure 9

BLOOD CULTURES

1. Full aseptic technique
   Mask and gloves worn

2. Tourniquet applied by assistant
   Skin carefully cleansed

3. Skin traction by left hand
   Needle inserted using right hand

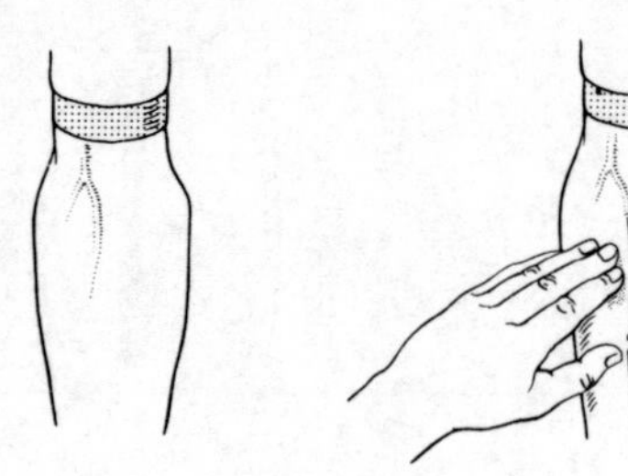

4. Needle and syringe removed
   Swab applied by assistant

5. Culture bottles filled, separate needles used

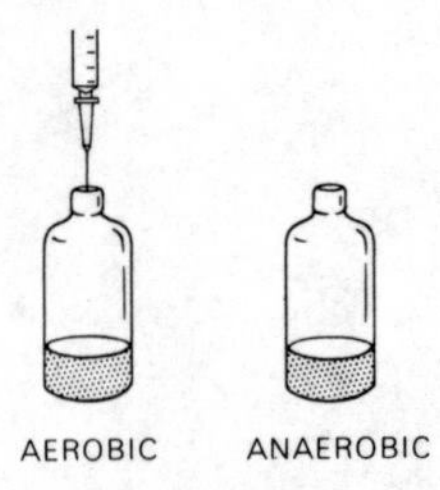

6. BLOOD CULTURES TAKEN TO LABORATORY IMMEDIATELY

Figure 10

is inserted by a single stab into a vein, in the manner previously described, using the left hand to give counter-traction to the skin. Twenty ml of blood is then withdrawn and the tourniquet removed by the assistant. The needle is then removed, the assistant being ready to press on the vein as soon as the needle is completely withdrawn.

The tops of the culture bottles should be cleaned with an antiseptic. The needle of the syringe is then changed, separate needles being used to inject the blood into the aerobic and anaerobic bottles. There is often a vacuum in these bottles and it is easy to inject the whole syringeful into one bottle unless this possibility is borne in mind. These bottles should be taken immediately to the Bacteriology Laboratory or placed in an incubator at 37°C.

5. TECHNIQUES FOR INTRAVENOUS INFUSIONS

Intravenous fluids are frequently used to maintain the fluid balance in patients who are unable to drink, or as a supplement to oral fluids. Blood and blood substitutes are given intravenously and solutions for parenteral nutrition by the intravenous route are now available. When indwelling intravenous cannulae are to be used, the hands should be thoroughly washed, and the nails scrubbed. A mask should be worn. A strict aseptic technique must be employed since introduction of bacteria may result in bacteraemia or suppurative thrombophlebitis with very serious consequences.

Equipment required

It is usual to have an assistant to help with the setting up of a 'drip'. The procedure can be greatly simplified by having all equipment available before starting.

1. A bottle of normal saline and an intravenous-giving set ready filled. Even though the drip is to be used for giving blood it is useful to start with saline since any accidents in setting up the 'drip' will not result in the wastage or spillage of blood.

2. Intravenous cannulae of your choice. Always have at least two available.

3. Sterile swabs, antiseptic solution and forceps, together with tourniquet or sphygmomanometer. A knife handle and sterile blade may be required for preliminary incision of the skin in some cases.

4. Adhesive tape ready cut, at least four strips of a good length being available. Bandages or netting, and a splint. In an emergency, the box containing the drip set may be used as a splint.

5. If a local anaesthetic is to be used, syringes, needles and local anaesthetic solution will be required. Syringe and specimen tubes should be available if blood sampling is to be performed at the same time.

Preparation of the patient

The procedure is first explained to the patient. The insertion of an intravenous cannula can be a painful procedure and the patient may feel that he is seriously ill and requires drastic treatment. Explain the function of the 'drip' Having selected a suitable site, the skin is thoroughly cleaned using sterile forceps to hold the swabs.

Local anaesthesia

This can be very useful especially if the patient is nervous or if the cannula to be inserted is large. A fine needle is inserted intradermally after preparing the skin and a bleb of local anaesthetic solution is raised over the proposed site of cannulation. A suitable anaesthetic is 1 per cent lignocaine, 0.2 to 0.5 ml being required. (Adrenaline in the local anaesthetic solution should not be used.) The bleb is then gently massaged into the skin and anaesthesia becomes effective within 1 minute. With many of the cannulae now available local anaesthesia is unnecessary. The needles are usually very sharp and cause a minimum of discomfort.

The equipment (Figure 11)

1. Most intravenous cannulae now consist of an outer non-irritant plastic cannula with central needle. Various lengths, sizes and shapes are available but, in general, the largest possible cannula should be used to ensure an adequate flow. Cannulae with an outer needle and inner plastic catheter are not recommended as the needles have been known to cut the cannulae which have disappeared into the circulation.

2. Intravenous giving sets are available as disposable units and are of two types. The first is for blood and blood products and has two chambers. The upper chamber contains a plastic gauze, which removes any clot that has formed. The lower chamber contains a plastic ball which acts as a valve when this chamber is full. Blood can therefore be pumped, using the hand, from this chamber into the patient by virtue of the ball valve. The second type of giving set is for non-sanguinous solutions and has a single chamber.

EQUIPMENT FOR INTRAVENOUS INFUSIONS

CANNULAE

Inner needle
Outer cannula

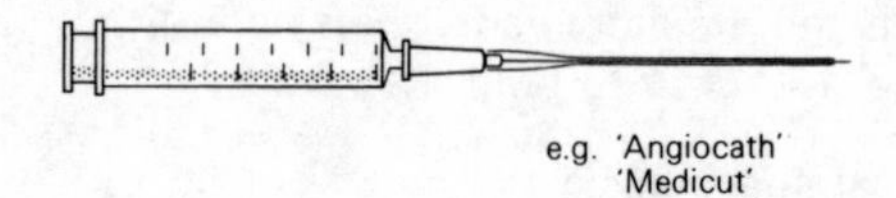

e.g. 'Angiocath'
'Medicut'
'Braunula'

Cannula with separate site for injections

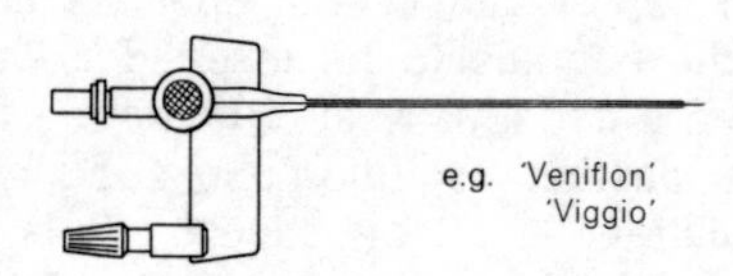

e.g. 'Veniflon'
'Viggio'

BUTTERFLY NEEDLE (Abbott Labs.)

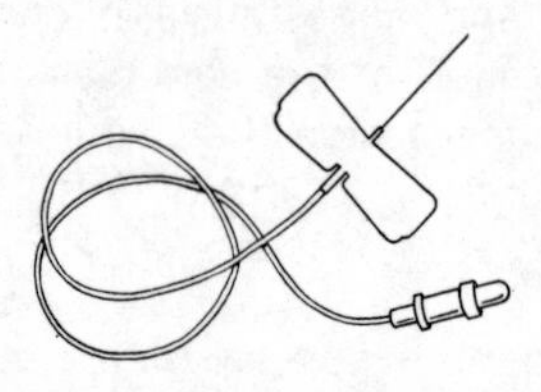

INTRAVENOUS GIVING SETS

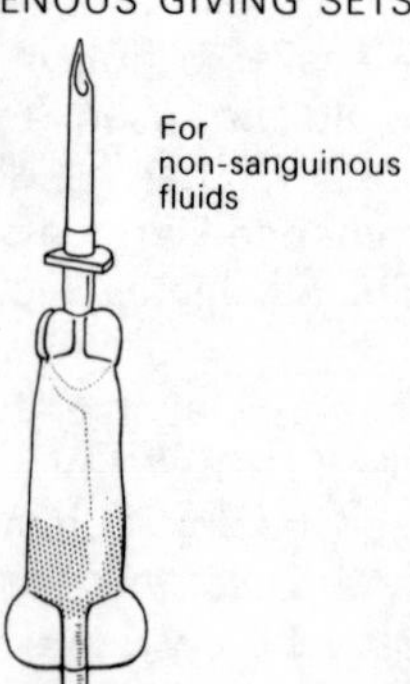

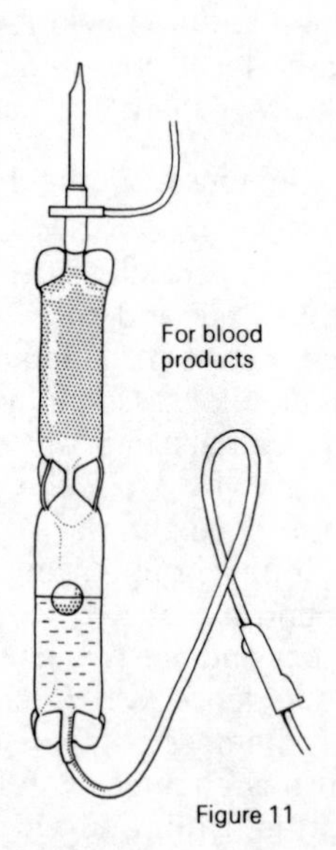

Figure 11

The method (Figure 12)

The technique for the insertion of an intravenous cannula is essentially the same as insertion of a needle for venepuncture. If the skin is thick and local anaesthetic has been used a small incision with a knife blade will facilitate insertion of the cannula. The needle and cannula are usually attached to a syringe for convenience and the needle is inserted obliquely through the skin and the vein entered. When this has been achieved, blood will be seen tracking up the cannula. Without inserting the needle further the plastic outer cannula is pushed gently into the vein. The needle is then removed and the cannula attached to the giving set. The intravenous infusion can then be commenced and if the cannula has been inserted correctly the flow should be even and rapid. The rate of the infusion is then adjusted as required.

Strips of adhesive tape are used to fix the cannula and 'drip' set tubing. If the cannula has been placed in the antecubital fossa, a splint is required to keep the elbow extended otherwise the cannula may kink or pierce the vein.

Sites for insertion of intravenous cannulae

The ante-cubital fossa. This is in many ways the easiest site for insertion of cannulae, but because splintage is required, mobility of the arm is reduced.

The forearm veins. The cephalic vein at the level of the radial styloid which, when the forearm is pronated and the hand pulled into ulnar deviation, is very suitable for cannulation. Splintage is not usually necessary and the patient can therefore move the arm freely.

Veins of the dorsum of the hand. These are again useful since mobility of the limb is retained. For arm veins it is a general principle that the most distal vein is used first, so that the proximal veins are preserved for future use.

The use of the external and internal jugular veins and the subclavian vein for intravenous cannulation will be discussed later under central venous pressure measurement.

METHOD OF INSERTING INTRAVENOUS CANNULAE

1. Tourniquet applied and skin cleansed
Needle with surrounding cannula inserted into a vein

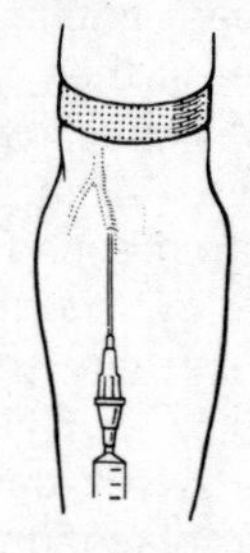

2. Tourniquet released
Cannula gently inserted further into the vein

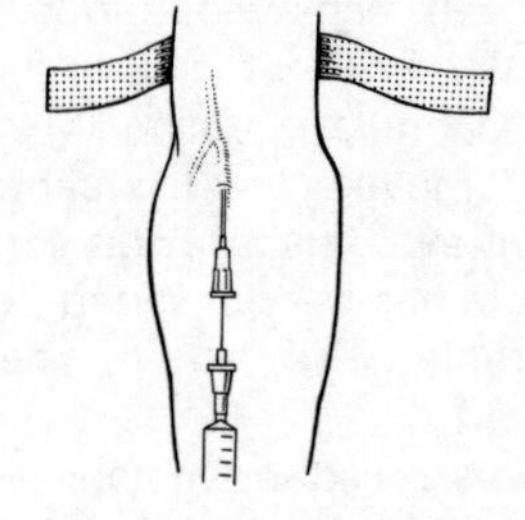

3. Drip set connected and infusion begun

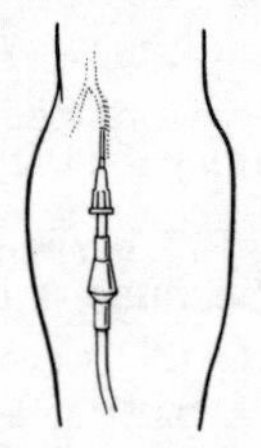

4. Cannula and infusion tubing taped in place

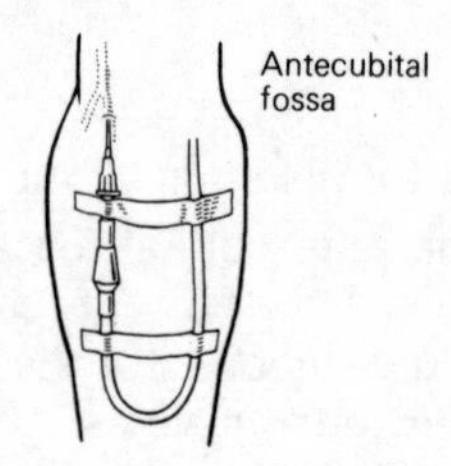

Dorsum of hand

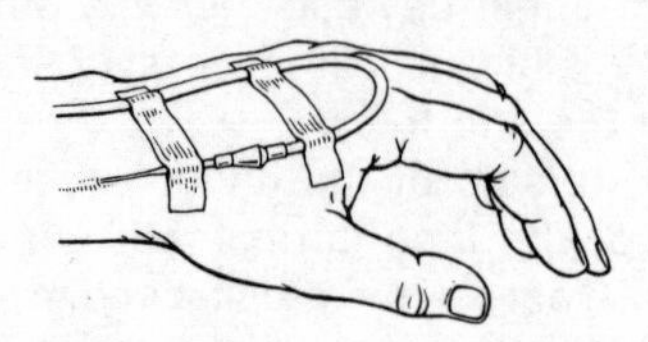

Figure 12

Difficulty with intravenous infusions

Once again, if difficulties are encountered, ask for help before damaging other accessible veins.

Obese patients. As with the venepuncture, patience, palpation and correct pressure are the secrets of success. Very often the site of a previous successful venepuncture gives a clue.

Hypotensive patients. The sphygmomanometer is a most useful instrument. Always allow adequate time for the veins to fill and ensure that good lighting is available. Palpate the veins prior to cannulation.

The patient with 'no veins'. Although this situation is unlikely to occur, the house surgeon may feel that this is the case with some patients. When a suitable vein cannot be found, there are several courses of action.

1. Ask someone else to have a look. A fresh eye often detects the vein you have missed.
2. Go systematically through the sites of venepuncture both looking and feeling. Use a sphygmomanometer.
3. In an emergency, an ordinary 20 gauge needle may be inserted into a small vein and enough fluid pumped through this to maintain life.
4. A cut-down may be required (See page 36).
5. Other sites such as the jugular or subclavian veins may be used (See page 42).

The rapid infusion of intravenous fluids (Figure 13)

It may often be necessary to give intravenous fluids rapidly to maintain life. Various solutions, from simple electrolyte infusions to blood or blood substitutes may be used. The first essential is that a large cannula is inserted into a large vein. By doubling the size of cannula the flow rate can be increased 16 times, whereas increasing the head of pressure to four times normal will only double the flow rate. Blood or fluid may be given rapidly either by pumping the lower chamber of a blood transfusion giving set, or by the use of a Martin's pump. The drip set tubing is threaded through the rollers of the pump and the handle rotated to increase the rate of fluid replacement. If large amounts of

RAPID FLUID REPLACEMENT

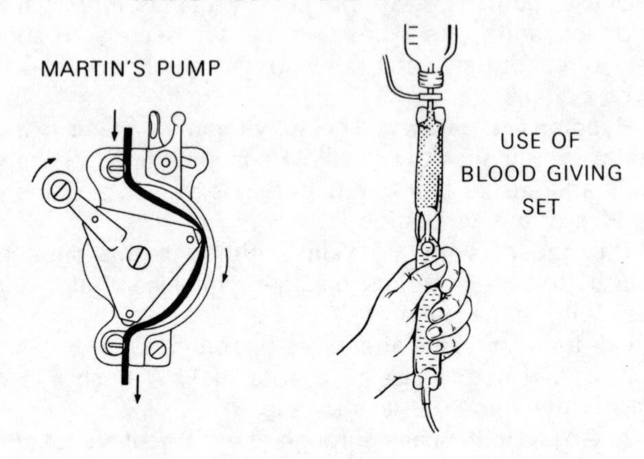

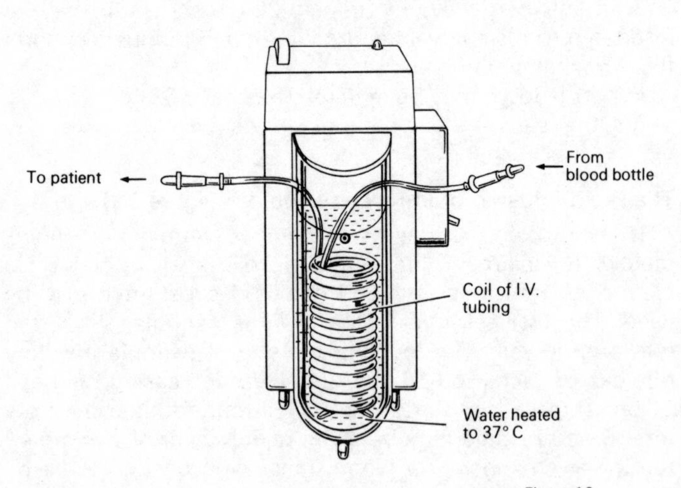

Figure 13

stored blood are to be given rapidly the temperature of the blood should be raised. This can be done by first circulating the blood through a blood warmer which consists of a length of intravenous tubing placed in a bath of pre-warmed fluid at 37°C. 50 mEq of sodium bicarbonate (50 ml of 8.4 per cent solution) should be given for every three litres of blood to correct for the acidosis of stored, anticoagulated blood.

Ten ml of 10 per cent calcium gluconate intravenously may be necessary to correct for the chelating action of the citrate anticoagulant, but its use is associated with cardiac irregularities, and so it should be used with caution. It must always be given slowly with E.C.G. monitoring. It should not be used where less than 3 litres of blood have been given.

'Drip' failure

The house surgeon is frequently called upon by the nursing staff to adjust the rate of intravenous fluids or to restart a blocked drip. On initial inspection it may be obvious that the drip is not working and that the arm is swollen and tender. In this event the cannula has probably pierced the vein and the fluid has been infused into the subcutaneous tissues. A 'tissued' drip must come down and, if intravenous fluids are still required, another one put up. If the arm is inflamed, then the cannula tip should be sent for bacteriological examination. If the drip has not tissued, go through the following sequence.

1. Check that the drip has been fully opened and that there is nothing constricting the arm such as a sphygmomanometer cuff.

2. Inspect the site. If it is inflamed, is the vein tender, or is thrombophlebitis present? In either case the drip should be taken down immediately. Again send the cannula tip to the Bacteriology Department for culture.

3. If the site is not inflamed it is likely that the vein has clotted or is in spasm. If the clot is recent, it may be dislodged by gentle pressure from a syringe containing either saline or citrate solution. Pressure should be even and firm and only a small quantity of fluid should be used (less than 10 ml) because of the danger of embolism.

4. If the drip is just going slowly it is worth either flushing out the cannula with citrate solution or raising the bottle of intravenous fluid as high as possible.

THE VENOUS CUT-DOWN

In certain circumstances no intravenous sites are available for percutaneous insertion of cannulae. In these cases veins known to be present in a constant position may be used and, as it is usually necessary to expose the vein, the term 'cut-down' is used. The doctor prepares as for the insertion of intravenous cannulae and in addition gloves and mask are worn. The procedure should be explained to the patient.

Equipment required

1. **Instruments.** Many hospitals have cut-down packs ready sterilised containing all necessary instruments. If not, then a sterile knife and blade (size 22), three pairs of curved artery forceps, small scissors, needle holder and dissecting forceps are required.

2. **Cannulae.** These are available in sterile packets and several of varying lengths and diameters should be ready, the largest possible being inserted. Gauges 14 to 16 are most suitable, either 30 or 60 cm long.

3. **Ties.** Catgut ties (2/0 or 3/0 chromic) should be available as well as 3/0 atraumatic black silk stitches for the skin. These may be included in the standard 'cut-down' pack, so make sure that you know what is available before starting the procedure.

4. **Local anaesthetic.** One per cent lignocaine with a syringe and needles should be ready, together with swabs and antiseptic solution for cleaning the skin.

Long saphenous vein cut-down at the ankle (Figure 14)

The vein may be visible or may be hidden by fat. Prepare the skin with antiseptic solution and infiltrate the area over the vein which lies anterior and just proximal to the medial

LONG SAPHENOUS CUT-DOWN AT THE ANKLE

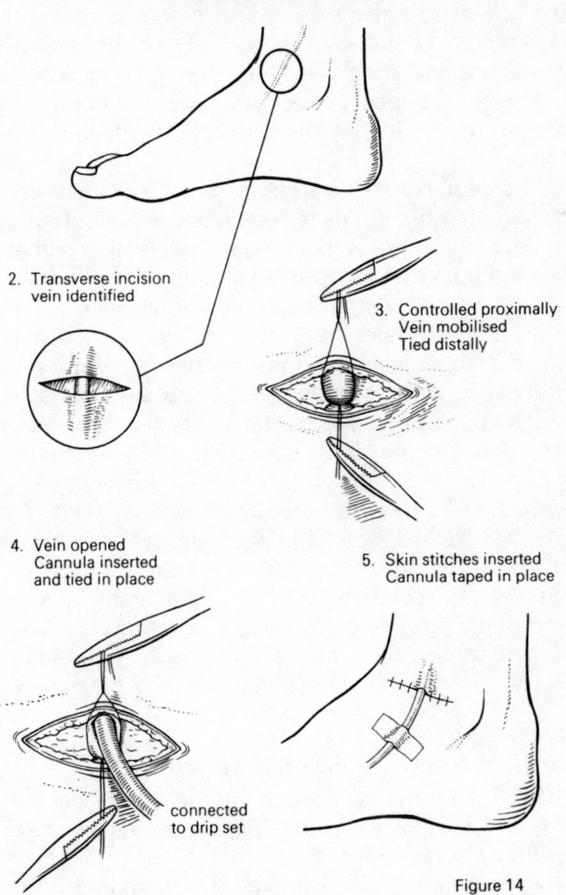

Figure 14

malleolus. Make a small transverse skin incision over the vein and dissect out the vessel using curved artery forceps. It is usually a fairly large structure and there is often a small vein close to it, and more superficial, which may mislead you.

Having found the vein pass artery forceps under it and pull through a double length of catgut having first separated the saphenous nerve from the vein. This catgut is then cut and the distal length tied around the vein. The ends are left long at this stage since they are useful for traction. The upper length of catgut is loosely tied and again held with forceps for traction. By pulling on the proximal tie bleeding can be controlled.

With the vein exposed a small 'v' is cut in its anterior wall making sure that the intima is completely divided. Using very fine forceps the vein is held open, while the catheter is inserted, the upper tie being momentarily relaxed to allow its insertion. The upper catgut tie is then firmly secured around the vein and catheter and the intravenous giving set connected. When inserting the catheter make sure that it enters the vein cleanly without stripping the intima. When the catheter is first inserted the flow may be poor initially so leave the drip running at full speed for a few moments. The skin is closed with 3/0 black silk, the cannula emerging from the wound. Alternatively the catheter may exit from a separate stab incision, distal to the main wound. A swab is placed over this and the catheter taped in place. The catheter can be removed later by withdrawing it from the vein and applying firm pressure to the area for one minute.

The method described above is the basic technique for all cut-down sites; the site of the initial skin incision alone varies.

Saphenous cut-down in the groin (Figure 15)

With this technique a catheter can be readily passed into the inferior vena cava so that large amounts of otherwise irritant fluids can be infused.

The skin of the groin is thoroughly prepared and local anaesthetic infiltrated 2 cm below the groin crease in its middle third. An incision is made along this line and, with

SITES FOR INTRAVENOUS CUTDOWNS

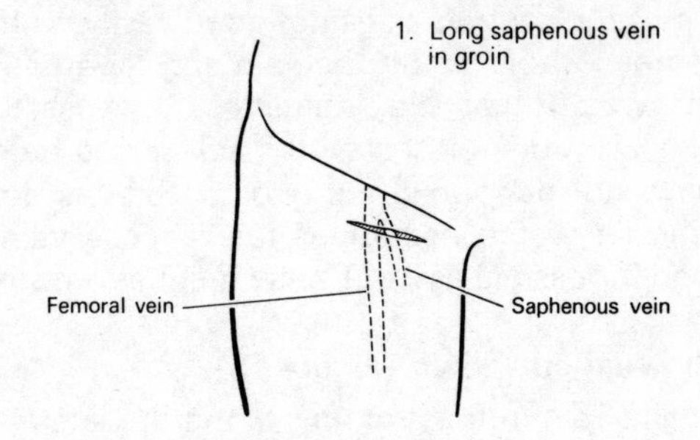

2. Cephalic vein in delto-pectoral groove

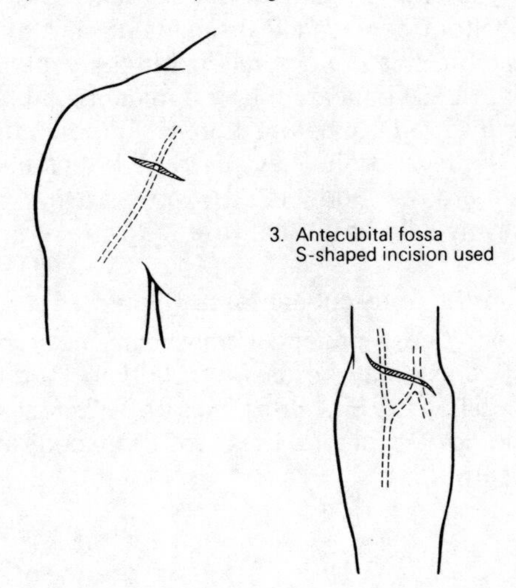

Figure 15

blunt dissection, the long saphenous vein identified. The veins in this region are inconstant and the first vein identified may not be the long saphenous vein. It should however communicate with the femoral vein. The vein is mobilised as before and the catheter inserted as far as possible and tied in place. If the cannula does not go in easily with gentle pressure, remove it and tie off the vein and try another one. Once again watch that the intima of the vessel is not stripped. The wound is closed with black silk as before.

If you have not performed the two procedures described then you should watch operations for varicose veins done in theatre and if possible assist. The techniques are similar.

The cephalic vein cut-down (Figure 15)

The cephalic vein in the arm runs along the lateral side of the upper arm between the biceps and brachialis muscle, then along the medial border of the deltoid muscle. This border of deltoid can readily be palpated and a transverse incision made in this region will enable the cephalic vein to be found. In obese patients the vein may be quite deep. The catheter is inserted as before but its introduction may be blocked at the level of the clavi-pectoral fascia. In this event the arm should be abducted by an assistant when the catheter can usually be further inserted.

Cut-down in the ante-cubital fossa (Figure 15)

In the very obese patient a transverse incision over the ante-cubital fossa may be useful in finding the cephalic or median cubital veins. Since this incision will cross the elbow joint it should be planned as an S-shaped incision to minimise scarring.

6. CENTRAL VENOUS PRESSURE MEASUREMENT

The measurement of the central venous pressure (CVP) is now regarded as an index of effective circulating blood volume. It is alternatively known as the right atrial pressure. The techniques for the insertion of a central venous pressure line are similar to venepuncture. Basically, a catheter is inserted by way of a peripheral vein into the great veins or the right atrium and, using this central venous line, the pressure within these veins is measured. The equipment required is similar to that required for an intravenous infusion. Before starting make sure that the central venous pressure giving set is full of fluid, and suitable catheters (at least two) are available. A centimetre scale will be required, together with a method for accurately relating the central venous manometer readings to a fixed point on the patient.

Method of insertion

For CVP measurement using a vein in the ante-cubital fossa the catheter should be 60 cm long. The most important feature is that the catheter should be placed in a large vein and advanced as far as possible. When other sites such as the jugular veins are used, shorter (30 cm) cannulae may be employed. The initial venepuncture in the ante-cubital fossa is made as before, the exact method used depending on the type of catheter employed (e.g. 'E-Z cath', 'Intramedicut' etc.).

At the end of this procedure, the fluid from the drip set should flow rapidly into the cannula and, if the great veins have been reached it is usual for fluid to leave the drip set bottle intermittently, the rate varying with respiration. If this does not occur then withdraw the cannula slightly in case the tip is located in a small venous branch. If this does not help then inject 2 ml of sterile citrate solution in case there is some clot within the catheter. The level which the catheter tip has reached can be assessed by comparing the length inserted with the stylet removed from the 'E-Z Cath.' or the plastic cover of the 'Intramedicut' or by subsequent chest X-ray.

Measurement of CVP (Figure 16)

The apparatus consists basically of a U-tube, one end of which is open to the air, the other being connected to a fluid reservoir. Using a three way tap either limb can be connected directly to the patient. To measure the CVP:

1. Fill the open limb of the U-tube using the three-way tap.
2. Connect the open limb directly with the patient.
3. If the catheter has been properly inserted and it is lying in the correct place, then the level of fluid should fall in a stepwise manner related to respiration. When the fluid has stopped falling, then the level should oscillate gently in time with respiration.
4. The final step is to relate the level of the fluid in the open limb to the pressure in the right atrium which, of course, varies depending on the position of the patient. To do this an arbitrary zero point is chosen. A number of these can be used but the most suitable is a point in the mid-axillary line representing the right atrium and this should be marked on the skin for reference. Alternatively, the angle of Louis may be chosen. A spirit level may be used to line up the reference point with the open limb, and using the moving scale marked in centimetres the zero mark is adjusted. A second method is to use a length of intravenous tubing, partially filled with water, which acts as a self-levelling manometer. One end is held at the reference point on the patient and the other at the open limb of the CVP manometer. The fluid level at this end of the intravenous tubing corresponds to the zero mark. The normal CVP varies considerably and of course depends on the reference point chosen. In general, values of +5 to +10 cm of water are within normal limits.

Use of the external jugular vein (Figure 17)

The external jugular vein may also be used both for intravenous therapy, and for central venous pressure

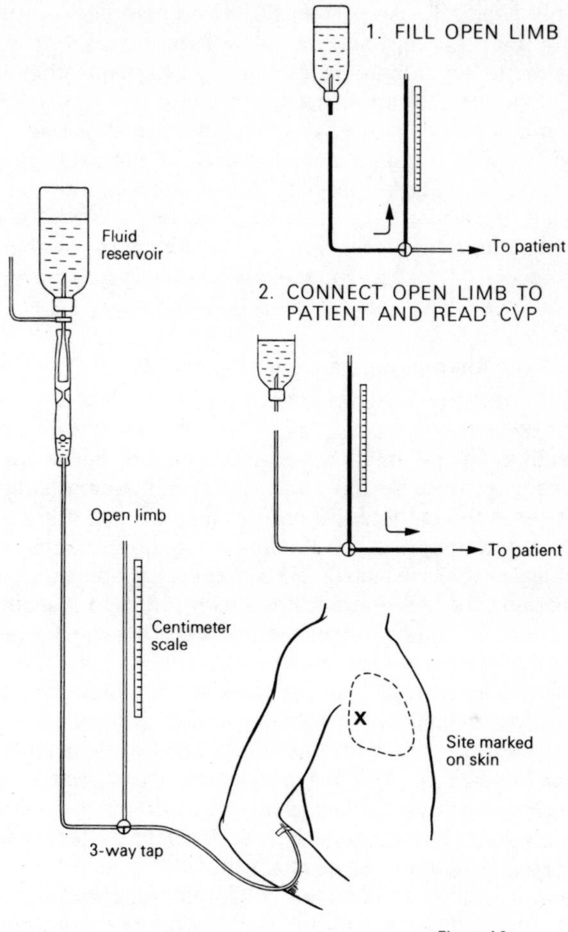
MEASUREMENT OF CENTRAL VENOUS PRESSURE
1. FILL OPEN LIMB
To patient
2. CONNECT OPEN LIMB TO PATIENT AND READ CVP
To patient
Fluid reservoir
Open limb
Centimeter scale
3-way tap
X
Site marked on skin

Figure 16

measurement. The patient is placed in the Trendelenburg (head down) position to distend the vein and prevent air embolism. If the vein is visible, then direct percutaneous puncture may be used. A 30 cm catheter (14 gauge) with internal needle is used. The needle and cannula are inserted directly into the vein and blood aspirated to confirm correct placement. The catheter is then gently inserted further and as rapidly as possible connected to the drip set. In some cases the catheter does not easily enter the superior vena cava, either because it enters a small branch of the vein or cannot negotiate the subclavian vein. If this occurs force must not be used or perforation of the vein may occur. After insertion of the catheter, if oscillation of the fluid level in the open limb occurs in relation to respiration, then it may be used to measure the CVP.

Use of the internal jugular vein (Figure 17)

This procedure is potentially very dangerous and should be performed only under supervision of an expert in the technique. The position of the internal jugular vein is constant and can be used for long term intravenous cannulation. In most cases the catheterisation may also be used for a central venous pressure line. A 30 cm (14 gauge) cannula with internal needle is used. The patient is placed in the Trendelenburg position and the head turned to the opposite side from the proposed venepuncture. The vein is located under the sternomastoid muscle. After thoroughly cleansing the skin and with full aseptic precautions including mask, gloves and gown, the needle is inserted at the outer border of the sternomastoid muscle 3 cm above the clavicle and driven inwards in the direction of the suprasternal notch. Aspiration will yield dark venous blood if the vein has been entered. The catheter is then inserted as the needle is withdrawn. As soon as possible this is connected to a drip set and infusion commenced. This catheter can be used for intravenous infusions, central venous pressure measurement, or for the sampling of venous blood.

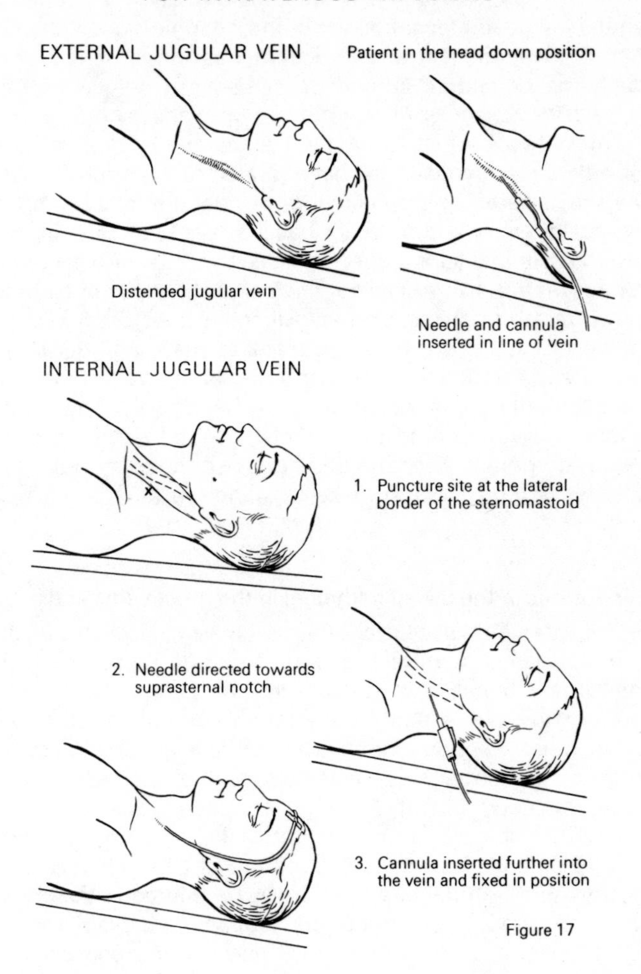
USE OF THE JUGULAR VEINS
FOR INTRAVENOUS INFUSIONS
EXTERNAL JUGULAR VEIN
Patient in the head down position
Distended jugular vein
Needle and cannula
inserted in line of vein
INTERNAL JUGULAR VEIN
1. Puncture site at the lateral
border of the sternomastoid
2. Needle directed towards
suprasternal notch
3. Cannula inserted further into
the vein and fixed in position

Figure 17

Subclavian vein puncture (Figure 18)

This vein may be used for long-term catheterisation for intravenous therapy, or central venous pressure measurement. The procedure is subject to more risks than internal jugular vein catheterisation including pneumothorax, haemothorax, air embolism and subcutaneous emphysema. Once again the procedure should be carried out only under the supervision of someone who is expert in the technique.

The patient is placed in the Trendelenburg position, the shoulders elevated, and the head rotated to the opposite side. The skin is carefully prepared and the operator fully scrubbed, gloved, gowned and masked. Local anaesthetic is infiltrated into the skin and subcutaneous tissue over the mid-point and inferior border of the clavicle. The needle of a 30 cm catheter is inserted through the skin and directed towards the suprasternal notch. To this end it is useful to place a finger in the suprasternal notch to help with orientation. When the vein has been entered, blood should flow back freely. The needle is then withdrawn and the catheter pushed gently into the vein and connected to the drip set as soon as possible. The catheter is then fixed in place by adhesive tape or a single stitch.

Precautions in the use of catheters in the great veins and heart

Measurement of central venous pressure and the ability to infuse large quantities of fluid into the great veins are undoubted benefits in many clinical situations. Several dangers however should be borne in mind. Firstly, catheters in the great veins are often used for the administration of drugs and it should be remembered that such drugs will reach the heart directly, in high concentrations. Solutions containing potassium or calcium salts, and drugs acting directly on the heart should therefore not be given by this means. Although the compound may be diluted in the giving solution, should the fluid be infused quickly, serious arrhythmias or even cardiac arrest can occur. Secondly, the heart may be ruptured by the catheter and this should be considered in any patient who has a central venous pressure

USE OF THE SUBCLAVIAN VEIN FOR INTRAVENOUS THERAPY

1. The relationship of the subclavian vein to the clavicle

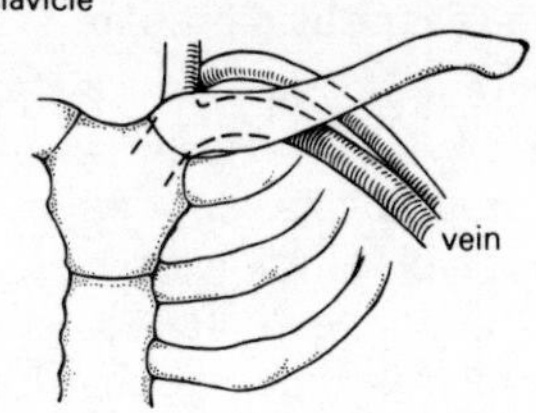

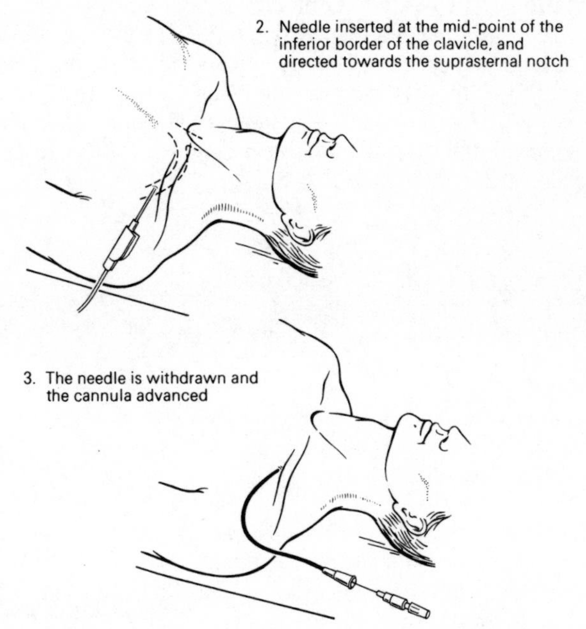

2. Needle inserted at the mid-point of the inferior border of the clavicle, and directed towards the suprasternal notch

3. The needle is withdrawn and the cannula advanced

Figure 18

line in position and whose condition deteriorates suddenly. A chest X-ray may show enlargement of the heart shadow due to the fluid in the pericardium.

Care of long-term intravenous cannulae

The puncture site should be inspected daily and signs of inflammation noted. A small amount of antibacterial cream may be smeared around the site each day. If signs of inflammation, redness or tenderness over the vein appear, then the catheter should be removed as soon as possible since thrombophlebitis may supervene. The catheter tip, and a swab of the puncture site should always be sent for bacteriological examination, and blood cultures should be taken in case bacteraemia is present. For long-term infusion of solutions containing large particles, or where frequent changing or modification of the infusion fluid may lead to a potentially contaminated infusate, an 'in-line' filter may be incorporated at the end of the giving set tubing to remove such particles or bacteria.

7. ARTERIAL BLOOD SAMPLING

Arterial blood sampling is required predominantly for the measurement of the pH of blood and for blood gas analysis. There are basically two methods by which arterial blood can be collected. The first method involves direct arterial puncture and is useful if a limited number of blood samples are required. The second method uses an indwelling arterial line and is required if the patient is seriously ill and multiple arterial blood sampling is necessary.

Direct arterial puncture

Only a few arteries are suitable for direct percutaneous puncture: the radial at the wrist, the brachial artery in the ante-cubital fossa, and the femoral artery in the groin. The femoral artery is of course the largest of the three and the easiest to puncture. In many patients, however, the femoral artery is atheromatous and needling may be sufficient to dislodge a plaque of atheroma or cause thrombus formation. For this reason the femoral artery should be used only when no others are available. The brachial artery is easy to palpate but any damage to the artery as a result of the needle puncture may result in severe ischaemia of the arm. For this reason the radial artery should be used in most cases.

When arterial blood is required, the blood sample has to be heparinised. To do this draw up into the syringe about 1 ml heparin (5,000 units/ml), clear all air bubbles then expel the heparin completely. This will leave a small amount of heparin in the syringe which will be sufficient for 10 ml of blood and will not dilute the specimen or, since heparin is a highly acidic compound, alters its pH. It is very important that no residual air is left in the syringe since this will equilibrate with the gases in the blood sample and invalidate blood gas analysis. If the sample is for blood gas analysis telephone the laboratory before the sample is taken to ensure that the equipment for measurement is ready for immediate use.

Methods of direct arterial puncture (Figure 19)

The hands are first thoroughly washed and the skin over the radial artery at the wrist cleaned in the usual way and a small quantity of local anaesthetic (1 per cent without adrenaline) is inserted over the proposed site of puncture. With the forefinger and middle finger of the left hand the artery is palpated. The fingers are then separated leaving a space of about 1 cm between them. The syringe is held vertically in the right hand, and the needle (20 gauge) is inserted through the skin and into the artery. When the arterial wall has been pierced, a small spurt of blood is often seen in the syringe. If the syringe is all-glass then arterial pressure alone will be sufficient to boost the plunger of the syringe. This is a useful check that the blood sample is arterial. With plastic syringes this does not occur to the same extent and the plunger may require to be withdrawn before blood is obtained. After sampling has been completed the needle is rapidly removed and a swab immediately pressed firmly over the needle mark by an assistant. This swab is held firmly in position for at least five minutes by which time the bleeding should have stopped. When the syringe is removed, it is rotated gently to mix the heparin and the blood. The sample is then taken immediately to the laboratory or is placed on ice until measurements can be performed. If this technique is performed expertly then multiple blood samples can be taken from the one artery.

The brachial artery in the ante-cubital fossa is readily palpable and arterial puncture is carried out in the manner described above. To obtain blood from the femoral artery, the procedure adopted is similar to that described above. The femoral artery in the groin is palpated (*see* Fig. 9) and, as with the femoral vein stab, the needle is inserted vertically through the skin into the femoral artery. In some cases a branch of the femoral vein lies deep to the femoral artery, and if the needle is inserted too deeply a mixture of venous and arterial blood may be obtained, making blood gas analysis unreliable. It is important therefore not to overshoot the artery.

DIRECT ARTERIAL PUNCTURE

RIGHT RADIAL ARTERY

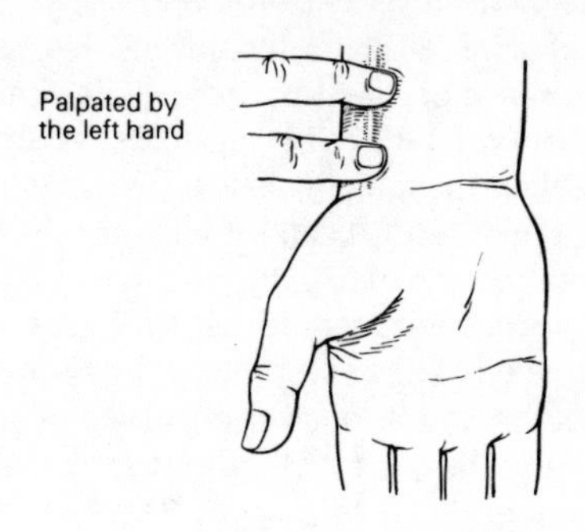

1. Syringe heparinised

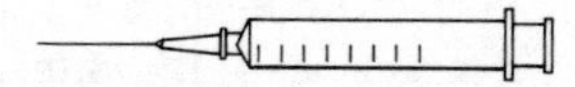

2. Needle inserted vertically into the artery

3. Needle removed and swab pressed over the puncture site

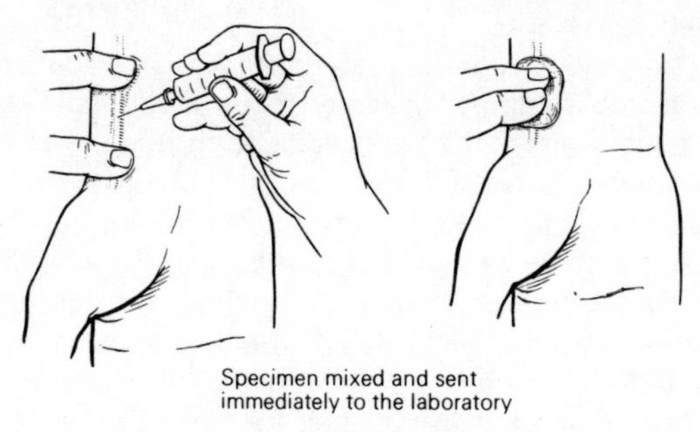

Specimen mixed and sent immediately to the laboratory

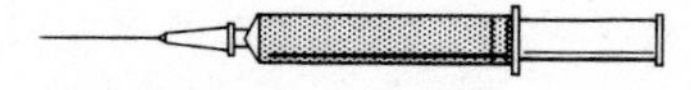

Figure 19

Radial artery cannulation for long-term sampling

Make sure before starting that all equipment is available and that suitable catheters are ready. Under local anaesthesia a small longitudinal incision is made over the radial artery at the wrist. In right-handed patients, the left hand should be used preferentially so that mobility of the arm is not restricted during the period of arterial catheterisation. The artery is identified and the vessel mobilised by gentle dissection. It is then controlled above and below by ligatures. A small nick is made in the vessel with sharp scissors and the catheter (14 to 16 gauge) 30 cm in length is then very gently inserted. After mobilisation the artery may narrow considerably and dilation of the vessel with fine artery forceps may be required. Great care should be taken not to strip the intima while doing this. Once the catheter has been inserted bleeding must be controlled either by inserting a small spigot into the end of the cannula, or by attaching a three-way tap turned to the appropriate off position. The cannula is tied in place and the skin closed with black silk. A short intravenous cannula with internal needle may also be used, the artery being directly punctured. Ligatures are not usually required and the skin is simply closed, the cannula being kept in place by a three-way tap taped to the skin.

The three-way tap is most useful in the collection of arterial blood samples, provided it is adequately cared for. Before taking blood, the tap is washed through with 1 to 2 ml of heparinised saline (5,000 units/500 ml). A syringe is then attached and 2 to 3 ml of blood withdrawn and discarded. The blood sample required is withdrawn. Finally, 0.5 ml of heparinised saline is inserted and the tap closed. With adequate care such an arterial line will remain patent for several days. To remove the catheter it is withdrawn and firm pressure applied to the area for five minutes.

Brachial artery cannulation for long-term sampling

It is important that only persons with considerable experience should use this artery for long term cannulation. The dangers may be minimal in experienced hands but may be considerable if great care is not taken. Thrombosis of the artery may result in severe ischaemia of the arm.

The technique used is a modification of the Seldinger technique for percutaneous cannulation of arteries. The arm is first extended fully, and the ante-cubital fossa thoroughly cleaned. A small amount of local anaesthetic (1 per cent without adrenaline) is infiltrated over the artery. While the local anaesthetic is taking effect the instruments are checked. A Courand or Riley needle is used and the nylon guide wire should fit snugly into the needle. A small incision (2 to 3 mm) is made in the skin to facilitate the penetration of the needle. The needle is then inserted into the artery, and it is usual to penetrate the back wall of the artery during this manoeuvre. The stilette is withdrawn slightly, as is the needle, until free pulsation of arterial blood occurs. At this point arterial bleeding is controlled by proximal pressure, the stilette removed, and the nylon guide wire inserted into the artery. The needle is completely removed and the catheter inserted into the artery with the aid of the guide wire. As the guide wire is finally removed, the catheter is connected to a three-way tap.

A simpler method is to use a catheter with attached needle such as the Beckton, Dickinson 'Longdwel' catheter. The site of puncture is prepared as above and the needle inserted into the artery. The stilette and needle are partially withdrawn until good pulsation occurs when the catheter is inserted into the artery. The needle and stilette are then fully removed and replaced by a matched Teflon obturator which locks onto the end of the catheter and obviates the need for heparinisation.

To remove an indwelling brachial artery catheter it is withdrawn slowly while pressure over the site, sufficient to occlude the radial pulse, is applied. This pressure is maintained for 10 minutes then gradually released. If any bleeding occurs at this time pressure should be re-applied.

8. THE URINARY SYSTEM

THE COLLECTION OF URINE

In the collection of urine several points must be remembered. Firstly, if any form of instrumentation is to be used there must be strict asepsis at all times. Secondly, if the urine is being collected for bacteriological examination it is important that no antiseptic solution comes into contact with the urine. Thirdly, specimens for culture should be transported to the laboratory within one hour of collection.

Mid-stream specimens of urine

This is a method which is now generally used to collect specimens for bacteriological examination. The procedure varies a little between males and females. The principle of the method is that the patient first passes a quantity of urine into a bedpan. This urine will contain contaminating urethral material and is therefore discarded. The subsequent specimen should be free from contamination and represent a true bladder specimen.

Females. This procedure is usually carried out by a nurse who should wear a mask and gloves. The patient is placed on a bedpan, and the vulva swabbed with warm sterile saline, each swab being used once only and the patient asked to pass urine. Once the flow has started a sterile gallipot is placed into the stream of urine and a mid-stream specimen collected. The urine is then immediately transferred to a sterile bottle and sent to the laboratory.

Males. The foreskin is retracted and, with sterile saline, the glans is cleansed. The patient then passes urine and once the stream has started a sterile container is used to collect a mid-stream specimen.

Preservation of urine for bacteriological analysis

A specimen of urine taken for bacteriological analysis must be sent to the laboratory within one hour if accurate results are to be obtained. If this is not possible then the urine should be stored at 4°C until it is possible to transfer it to the laboratory. Recently a method of immediate plating of urine specimens has been described using a slide coated with culture medium placed in a sterile universal container ('Uricult'). The urine to be tested is added to the container and incubation of the specimen begun at once. This method is at present under evaluation.

CATHETERISATION OF THE BLADDER

This procedure may be required in order to obtain urine for bacteriological purposes or to relieve a retention of urine. The catheter may be inserted through the urethra or supra-pubically.

Types of catheter used (Figure 20)

Many types of catheter are available, only the commonest will be described here.

1. **Foley catheter.** A self retaining catheter kept in place by a balloon filled with saline. Note the volume of the fluid, marked on the catheter, required to fill the balloon.
2. **Malecot catheter.** Self retaining by virtue of its flanged ends. This catheter requires an introducer for insertion.
3. **Harris catheter.** More rigid than the above and not self retaining. The catheter is held in place either by tapes or, if inserted at operation, by sutures.
4. **Gibbon catheter.** A long catheter, available in small sizes specially suitable when prostatic obstruction is present.
5. **Whistle Tip and Coudee catheters.** The tips are modified for ease of insertion past a prostatic obstruction.

Urethral catheterisation in the male (Figure 21)

The procedure requires the utmost care and an aseptic technique. The procedure is fully explained to the patient before starting. The patient lies on his back with his legs apart and pubic area is then shaved. The doctor scrubs up and puts on mask and gloves. Sterile towels are laid around

TYPES OF URETHRAL CATHETER

FOLEY CATHETER

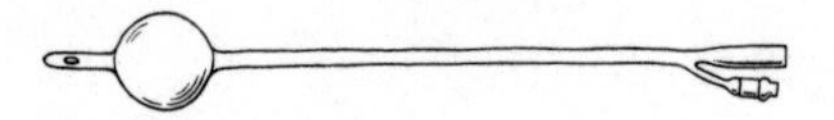

MALECOT CATHETER

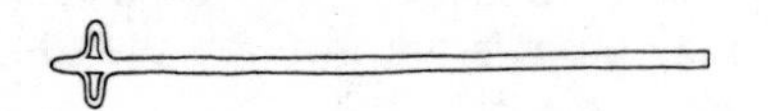

HARRIS CATHETER

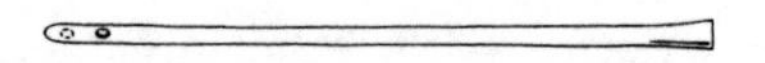

GIBBON CATHETER

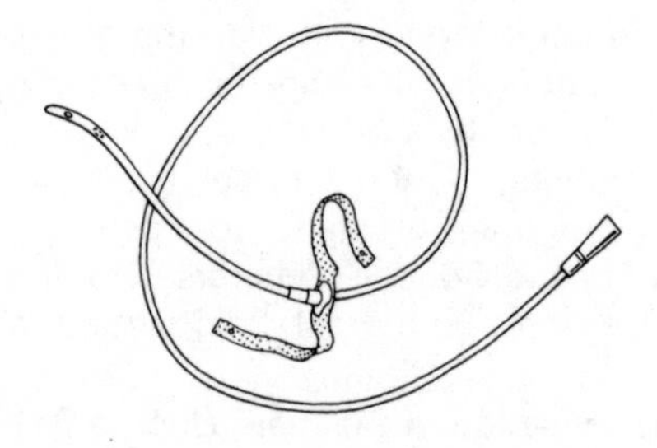

Figure 20

URETHRAL CATHETERISATION IN THE MALE

1. Strict asepsis, mask and gloves worn
2. Penis held in swab with left hand
   Patient towelled, the prepuce retracted
   and the glans cleaned

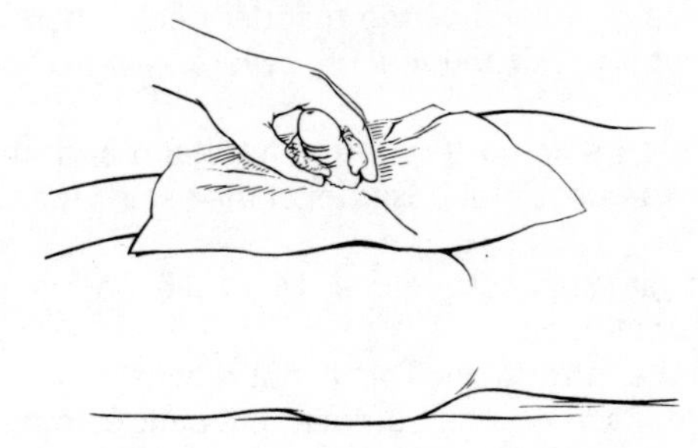

3. Ready lubricated catheter inserted
   with right hand using forceps

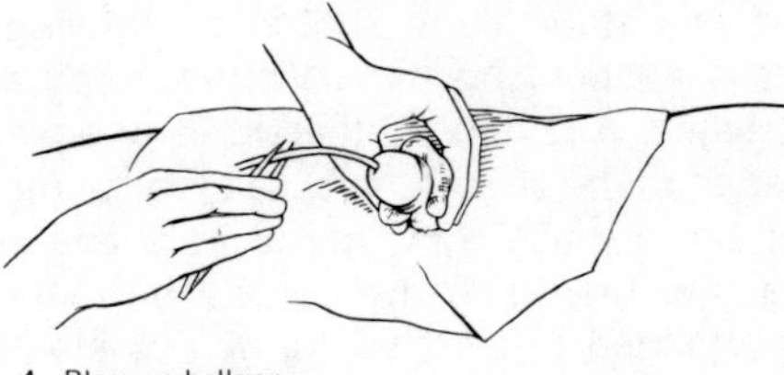

4. Blow up balloon
   and replace prepuce

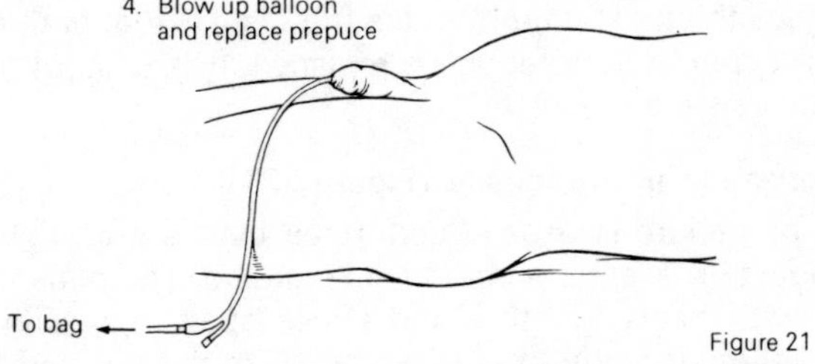

Figure 21

the penis, and over the anterior abdominal wall. Before starting make sure that the catheter (18 to 20 F.G.) is lubricated with sterile jelly and that a receptacle is in place to catch the urine. Soak a swab in chlorhexidine in water and holding it in the left hand retract the prepuce. In this way the left hand is kept as sterile as possible, the swab alone touching the patient. When the glans has been exposed, it is carefully washed using aqueous chlorhexidine on swabs held by forceps. The catheter is then gently inserted. Difficulty may occur at the level of the bladder neck where narrowing is not uncommon. If this occurs several manoeuvres may be tried.

1. Pull the penis tight with the left hand and move it from a vertical to a horizontal position, at the same time introducing the catheter.

2. Try a smaller catheter, a 14 or 16 gauge Foley or a Gibbon catheter.

3. Use the introducer. This is not meant to give additional force to the insertion of a catheter, but simply to make it more rigid. Once again move the penis from the vertical to the horizontal position while gently introducing the catheter. When the catheter has been inserted, the introducer is removed. At this stage urine should be flowing freely and the catheter is fixed in position. With a Foley catheter the balloon is inflated. A Gibbon catheter has two plastic flanges which are taped to the skin at the base of the penis. A Malecot catheter is held in place by virtue of its shape and a Harris catheter requires taping to the penis. The catheter is then spigoted or attached to a collecting bag by sterile tubing.

Perhaps the most important feature of all is that at the end of the procedure the prepuce is replaced. If this is not done, paraphimosis may result.

Catheterisation in the female (Figure 22)

This procedure is usually performed by the nursing staff. Once again an aseptic technique is required. The patient lies supine with heels together and knees apart, exposing the vulva. Adequate lighting is essential. With the left hand the labia are separated and using aqueous chlorhexidine or other

URETHRAL CATHETERISATION IN THE FEMALE

1. Mask and gloves are worn
2. Using forceps labia are cleansed

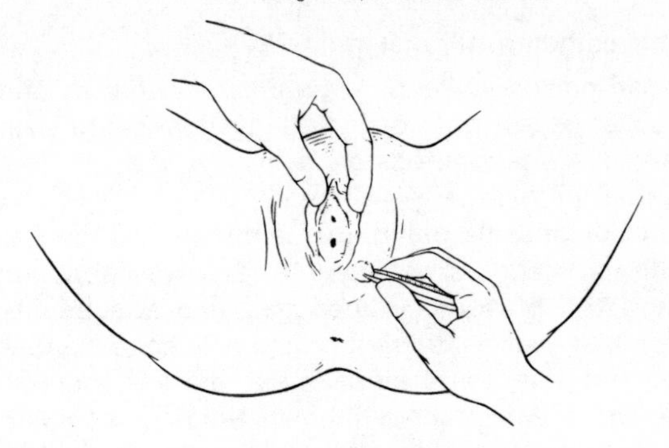

3. Urethral orifice identified
   Catheter inserted using forceps
   and balloon blown up

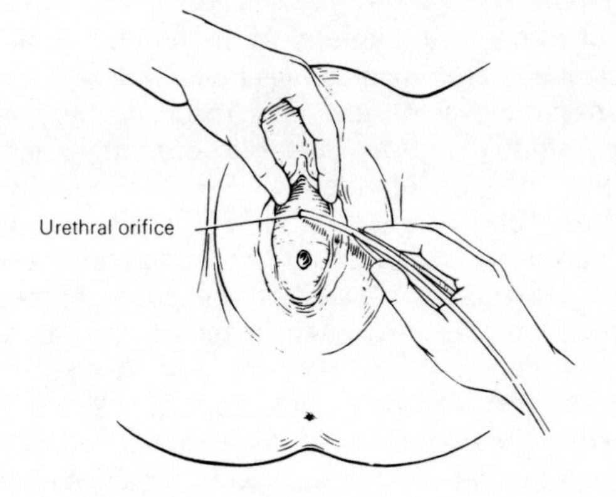

Figure 22

antiseptic solution, the labia are cleansed. Each swab is used once only and is held with forceps. The area should be swabbed from an anterior to a posterior direction to avoid perineal contamination. The urethral orifice is then identified and the already lubricated catheter (size 20 to 22) is inserted and fixed in place.

Suprapubic catheterisation (Figure 23)

This method of collecting urine is useful if urethral catheterisation is not possible or if long term catheterisation is anticipated. Three methods are available, in each case it is assumed that the bladder is distended.

1. **Use of disposable polythene cannulae.** This is useful if short term drainage is required. The lower abdomen is shaved and the bladder outlined palpated and percussed. The abdominal wall is then thoroughly cleaned and local anaesthetic infiltrated at a point in the mid-line 5 cm above the pubis. The needle of a polythene catheter is then plunged through skin, subcutaneous fat, linea alba and into the bladder. The stylet is then removed and urine drained via sterile tubing into a bag. It is fixed to the skin by a stitch or adhesive tape.

2. **Use of trocar and cannula.** As before, the abdomen is shaved, cleaned, and local anaesthetic infiltrated. With a knife, a small transverse incision is made in the skin 5 cm above the symphysis pubis just big enough to allow the trocar to enter the subcutaneous tissue. With a rotary movement the trocar and cannula are thrust into the bladder. This may be painful, not because of the instrument, since the tissues should be anaesthetised, but because of pressure on the bladder. With the instrument inserted, the trocar is removed and a finger placed over the end. A gush of urine usually occurs at this stage. A 20 to 24 F.G. Malecot catheter on an introducer is then inserted, the cannula and introducer removed, and the catheter connected to a bag. Within a few weeks a tract develops making it easy to replace and remove the catheter.

3. **Open procedure (Figure 24).** As before the area is shaved and cleaned. Local anaesthetic is infiltrated along a

SUPRAPUBIC CATHETERISATION OF THE BLADDER—I

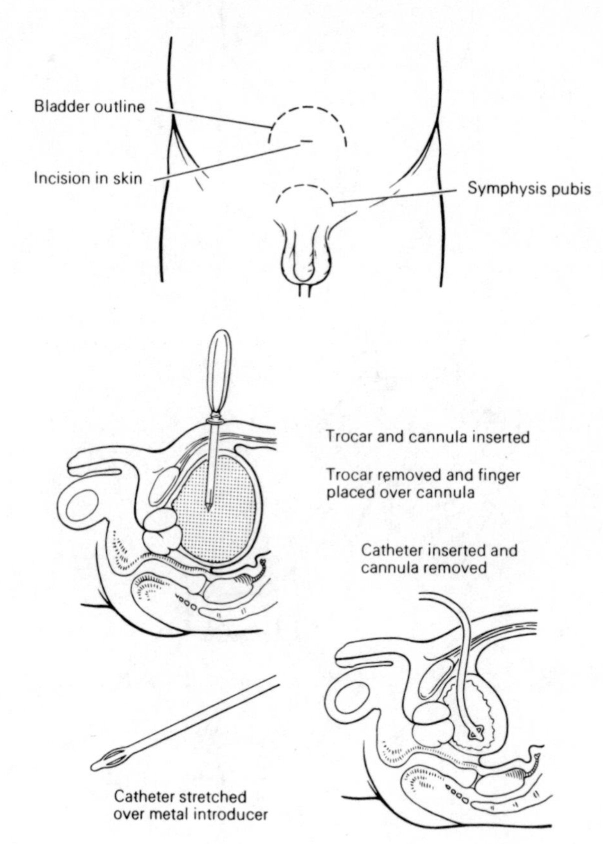

Figure 23

SUPRAPUBIC CATHETERISATION OF THE BLADDER—II

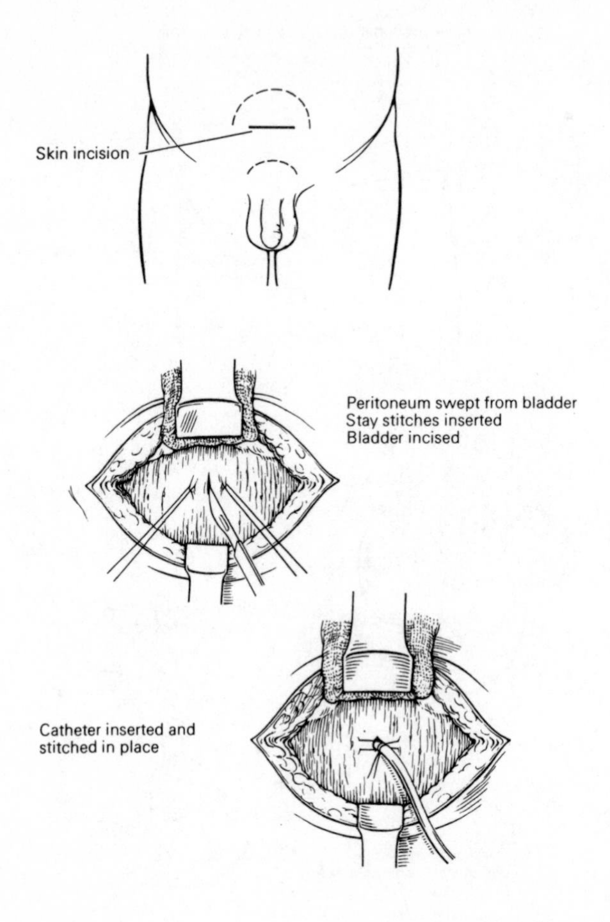

Figure 24

line 5 cm above the pubis, 5 cm long. Using a knife a transverse incision is made along this line and deepened to the muscle layer. This layer is incised vertically in the mid-line and the muscles separated. The peritoneum should, if the bladder is distended, be well out of the way at this point. It is important however to make sure that the peritoneum is swept clear of the bladder. The fascia overlying the bladder is then divided and the bladder wall identified. Two stay sutures of 2/0 catgut are inserted 1 cm apart, and the bladder opened. Suction should be available at this stage. A Foley or Malecot catheter is then inserted and the stay stitches tied around it. The superficial layers are then repaired with catgut and the skin closed with silk.

CYSTOSCOPY

This procedure may be performed under general or local anaesthesia. If general anaesthesia is to be used, the patient is prepared as described in Chapter 2. If it is proposed to carry out divided renal function tests following ureteric catheterisation it is usually necessary to give the patient intravenous fluids to maintain hydration and give an adequate urine volume.

The cystoscope is basically a telescope with a suitable means of lighting. An attachment is available in order that sterile fluid, saline or water, can be passed through the cystoscope into the bladder for distension or irrigation. There are many variations in cystoscopes and special types for retrograde catheterisation, biopsy and cautery have been designed. It is worthwhile before proceeding with cystoscopy to test the instrument, its lighting and attachments.

The procedure is essentially similar to urethral catherisation. Preliminary bouginage however may be necessary. The cystoscope is gently inserted, the weight of the instrument alone being of sufficient force. Warm fluid is then run into the bladder and a systematic examination carried out. Orientation is facilitated by identification of the ureteral orifices and the air bubble which is located under the anterior surface of the bladder. At the end of the procedure fluid and urine should be drained from the bladder.

Retrograde catheterisation of the ureters

Using a specially constructed cystoscope it is possible to pass fine catheters into the ureters for further examination of the renal tract. The cystoscope is passed as before and, after inspecting the bladder and localisation of the ureteral orifices, catheters are passed up the ureters with the use of an adjustable director located at the end of the cystoscope. At the end of the procedure it is important that this director is placed in line with the cystoscope so that no damage to the urethra results on removal of the instrument.

RENAL BIOPSY

This may be carried out under local or general anaesthesia. It may be performed either using a needle or as an open biopsy. In either case one litre of blood should be cross-matched and be available prior to biopsy. If local anaesthesia is to be used preliminary premedication is necessary (Chapter 2).

If an open biopsy is to be employed then a lumbar incision with direct visualisation of the lower pole of the kidney is used. The patient should be closely observed following the procedure in case of bleeding from the biopsy site. The pulse and the blood pressure are recorded half-hourly for 24 hours and the colour and volume of the urine noted.

Using the needle biopsy method either local or general anaesthesia may be employed. Preliminary radiology of the kidneys is usually necessary for accurate localisation and it is recommended that this should be performed at the time of the biopsy. The patient lies prone and the iliac crest, 12th rib, and the mid-line are marked on the back, together with the proposed biopsy site, which is usually over the lower pole of the kidney. This lies at the junction of the middle and outer thirds of a line between the tip of the last palpable rib and the mid-line. The skin and deeper tissues are then anaesthetised and the renal biopsy needle, in most cases a modification of the Vim-Silverman needle, is inserted. This is done in stages as the patient holds his breath. When the needle has been correctly inserted it should oscillate with respiration. The biopsy is taken while the patient holds his breath to ensure that laceration of the kidney does not occur. The needle is removed and the puncture mark sealed with adhesive spray and a dry dressing. The patient is closely observed for the following 24 hours in case bleeding occurs.

9. PROCEDURES ON THE GASTROINTESTINAL TRACT

NASOGASTRIC INTUBATION

The passage of a tube into the stomach is necessary for many purposes; gastric suction, gastric secretion tests, gastric lavage etc. It is usual to pass the tube via the nose but in certain cases it will be more convenient to pass the tube by mouth.

Before starting, the procedure should be fully explained to the patient. It is an unpleasant experience to have a naso-gastric tube passed and the patient should have as much encouragement and reassurance as possible. Have everything readily available; nasogastric tube, 16 to 20 gauge, ready lubricated, swabs, spigot or connecting tube, and containers for collecting gastric fluid. If gastric lavage is to be carried out, funnel, washing fluid and receptacle should be available.

Technique (Figure 25). The patient is comfortably propped up in bed and the nose inspected. It is often apparent that only one nostril can be used because of nasal deformity. The lubricated tube is then gently passed through the nose to the nasopharynx. At this stage the patient is asked to breathe in and out gently through the mouth. As the tube is gently inserted further the patient is then asked to swallow, and often a small amount of sterile water given at this time will assist swallowing. With patience, gentleness and persistence the tube will usually pass into the oesophagus and from there into the stomach. If this does not occur, then the tube should be removed, the patient reassured and the procedure repeated using a smaller diameter tube. It is usually a mistake to use a softer tube since this often curls up in the pharynx.

Some patients prefer to pass the tube themselves and they can often do this very successfully. In these cases it is usual to pass the tube through the mouth, and this is also so when the nasal passages are blocked.

It is usually easy to tell whether the tube is in the stomach or not, but certain confirmatory tests may be necessary.

PASSAGE OF NASOGASTRIC TUBE

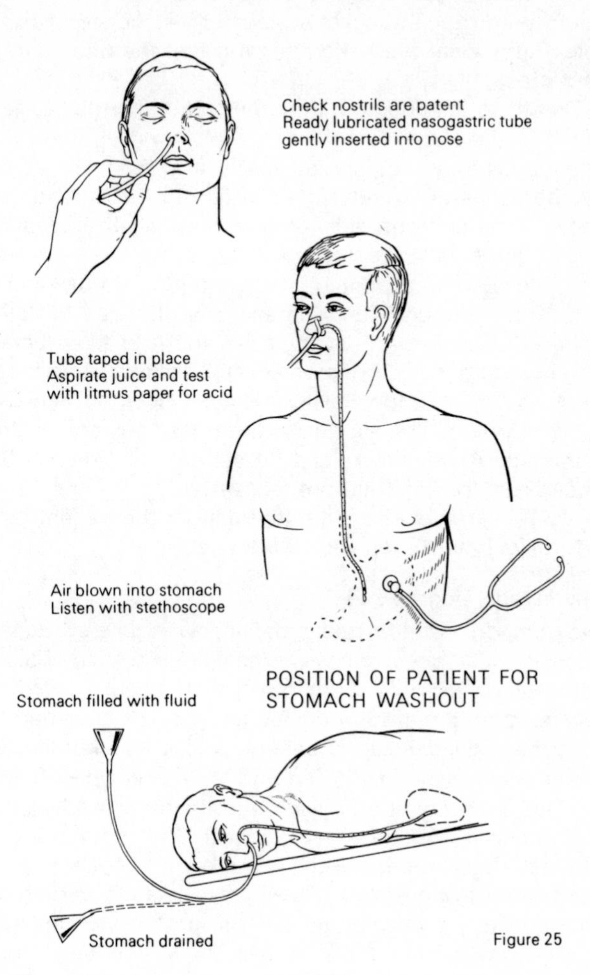

Figure 25

1. The stomach contents are aspirated and the character noted. The pH is tested using litmus paper and, if acid, the tube can be assumed to be in the stomach.

2. By blowing a small amount of air down the tube, listening with the stethoscope placed over the stomach will enable you to hear the air, confirming that the tube is in the correct place.

3. Breath sounds coming from the end of the tube suggest that it is in the trachea.

The tube is fixed in place by taping it to the nose, though it may be necessary to alter the position of the tube in order to aspirate the contents adequately; the position is changed by moving the tube gently upwards and downwards until gastric juice can be aspirated. To clear a blocked nasogastric tube a 50 ml syringe filled with saline is attached to its end and the fluid flushed down the tube and into the stomach. This may require to be done on several occasions, especially if there has been upper gastrointestinal haemorrhage with clotting of blood. The syringe is then used to aspirate from the stomach. Always remember to correct the patient's fluid balance chart for any fluid not recovered.

The tube is removed by gentle traction, the patient being asked to swallow during the withdrawal.

Gastric lavage (Figure 25)

The procedure is indicated in patients who have swallowed poisonous substances, or have taken an overdosage of drugs. It may also be used to wash out the stomach if there has been a prolonged period of gastric retention. It is carried out only in the fully conscious patient unless an endotracheal tube has been inserted. To the end of the nasogastric tube which has been correctly placed in the stomach a length of rubber tubing is attached, together with a filter-funnel. Have the lavage fluid ready, with a bucket for collecting the effluent. About one gallon of warm tap water is required in the adult. The patient should lie face down with the head over the edge of the table or bed, or in the head down position. Using this method of positioning the risk of inhalation of stomach contents is minimised. Initially 200 ml of fluid is passed into the tube and then into the stomach, the funnel is then placed below the level of the gastric content and allowed to drain into a separate bucket by a process of syphoning. This process is repeated until the gallon of water has been used.

Carefully examine the character of the fluid and keep a specimen of it for subsequent examination or analysis.

The gastrostomy tube

This tube may be used as an alternative to nasogastric suction, and a Foley catheter, balloon size 5 ml is the usual choice. It will of course have been inserted into the stomach at operation and anchored to it by an absorbable suture. It is usually removed 7 to 10 days after operation, and this is performed by gentle traction on the tube after first letting down the balloon and removing any skin stitches. If the tube cannot be readily removed, or its removal is causing pain, then the patient should be sedated before repeating the manoeuvre.

Some types of gastrostomy tubes, feeding gastrostomy tubes, have a triple lumen (Figure 26). One lumen is for gastric suction as with an ordinary gastrostomy tube; the second is for inflating the balloon to retain the gastrostomy tube in position; the third is fed into the duodenum or jejunum. The latter can be used as a feeding jejunostomy, fluid being passed from a drip set bottle into the upper part of the jejunum.

Gastric secretion tests

These are most commonly used for the pre- and post-operative assessment of patients suspected of having peptic ulceration. A nasogastric tube is passed as described, the patient having been fasted for 12 hours prior to the test. The position of the tube is critical and this is usually verified under radiological control. Basal samples of gastric juice are taken before the appropriate test is carried out. The volume of the sample, pH and acid concentration are measured, and the character of the gastric juice observed and the presence of bile noted. For the modified histamine test, 0.04 mg histamine acid phosphate/kg is given intramuscularly, the antihistamine mepyramine maleate (50 mg) being given 30 minutes beforehand to prevent side effects. Alternatively, pentagastrin (6 μg/kg) intramuscularly, without the antihistamine, may be given. The gastric juice is collected over 15 minute periods for two hours and the pH, volume and acid concentration measured.

The insulin test, used to assess vagal integrity is performed by giving 20 units of soluble insulin intravenously. This dose of insulin should be sufficient to reduce the blood sugar level to 40 mg per cent. Gastric juice is collected at 15 minute intervals over a period of two hours and the measurements detailed above are made. Close observation of the patient is necessary during this test for evidence of severe hypoglycaemia which is corrected if necessary by intravenous glucose. The interpretation of these tests is outwith the scope of this book.

THE STRING TEST

In the case of undiagnosed upper gastrointestinal bleeding, the string test or one of its modifications may be useful in finding the level of the bleeding and the house surgeon may be asked to perform it. Basically this test involves passing a string with internal markers into the upper gastrointestinal tract. A marker dye is then injected intravenously and is discharged at the site of the bleeding into the lumen of the gut and on to the string. The site is then detected by removing the string after radiologically determining that it has successfully negotiated the pylorus. The relation of the dye to the markers on the string can then be used to determine the site of bleeding.

The string can be constructed using fine cord such as that used for covering arterial instruments or a Rugby boot lace, and threading through this the radiologically opaque threads from Raytex swabs, suitably knotted at intervals as markers. The end is weighted with a small metal ball. After passing the string through the mouth and allowing it to negotiate the pylorus, the patient is given intravenously 10 ml of 10 per cent fluorescein solution which, it is hoped, will stain the string at the site of bleeding. Fluorescein can then be visualised under ultraviolet light after removal of the string. Such a test will only be useful if active bleeding is occurring and the use of selective superior mesenteric or coeliac artery angiography is more sophisticated and perhaps more reliable if the rate of bleeding is more than 10 ml/minute.

THE SENGSTAKEN TUBE (Figure 26)

This tube is used to control the bleeding from oesophageal varices. It is basically a triple lumen nasogastric tube with two balloons. The lower balloon is to locate the oesophageal-gastric junction and the proximal one to compress the varices. Before passing the tube make sure that the lumen is patent, that the ends of the tubes are clearly marked so that the correct balloon will be inflated and the volume to fill each balloon is known. The tube is then well lubricated and passed gently through the mouth into the stomach. When in the stomach the gastric, or distal balloon, is inflated with 100 to 150 ml of water and the tube gently withdrawn until the balloon is arrested at the gastro-oesophageal junction. This manoeuvre ensures that the longer oesophageal balloon now lies over the varices in the oesophagus. The oesophageal balloon is then inflated and the bleeding veins compressed. The oesophageal balloon may be inflated with fluid, 100 ml being required, or air. Using a sphygmomanometer, air is pumped into the oesophageal balloon until a pressure of 25 to 30 mm Hg is reached. It is necessary to maintain traction on the tube to retain the balloons in the correct position. The tube may be taped to the face, or 0·5 to 1 kg traction may be applied using a pulley. Pressure necrosis may occur with this tube so that it must be deflated after 24 hours.

LARGE BOWEL ENEMAS

A variety of solutions from soap and water to castor oil can be used for enema fluids. The technique however is the

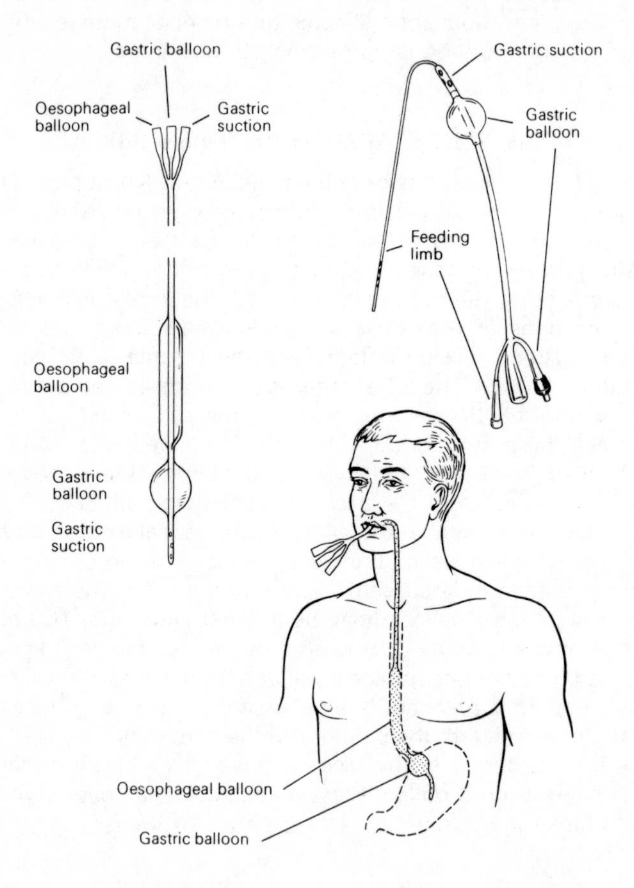
SENGSTAKEN TUBE
KAY'S FEEDING GASTROSTOMY TUBE
Gastric balloon
Oesophageal balloon
Gastric suction
Gastric suction
Gastric balloon
Feeding limb
Oesophageal balloon
Gastric balloon
Gastric suction
Oesophageal balloon
Gastric balloon

Figure 26

same in all cases. The patient is placed in the left lateral position and a towel and polythene sheet placed under the buttock. A wide bore catheter of soft material (12 EG) is attached to rubber tubing and a conical funnel. All air is expelled from the tubing, the catheter lubricated and inserted upwards and backwards into the rectum. Keeping the funnel at a constant level, 500 to 1000 ml of the fluid are inserted and the patient asked to retain the fluid in the rectum until there is a desire to defaecate. A commode or bed pan should be nearby so that the stool can be collected. After evacuation the stool is examined and a sample retained if required.

If the enema has been given for therapeutic purposes, such as in ulcerative colitis, and requires to be retained, the patient should have the procedure fully explained to him. Retention is aided by elevating the bed. A patient who requires an enema for this purpose can usually be taught to perform the procedure himself without difficulty.

The normal enema consists of soap and water, 600 to 1200 ml being given. If faecal impaction is present however, the stool may be softened by giving olive oil (100 to 200 ml) which is retained for 20 minutes. If effective the stool should become softer and a soap and water enema then given. This may require to be repeated daily for some days and if it fails then manual evacuation may be required.

Manual evacuation of faeces

This procedure is usually delegated to the most junior member of the surgical team. Nevertheless it remains a most important part in the management of certain patients. For the elderly patient with a lax anal sphincter, part of the procedure may be accomplished in the ward without a general anaesthetic. In patients where this does not apply, or is unsuccessful, general anaesthesia is required.

The patient is prepared for a general anaesthetic and, after anaesthesia has been induced, an endotracheal tube should be passed since the procedure may well induce laryngeal spasm. The patient is placed in the left lateral position. The doctor should wear gown, mask and gloves, for protective reasons only. It is also wise to wear operating theatre clothes and a pair of boots. The well lubricated hand is inserted and as much faeces as possible removed by the fingers. Solid portions of faeces which cannot otherwise be removed should be broken down by the fingers. If this is unsuccessful a flat instrument, traditionally a spoon, should be gently inserted into the rectum and used to break up the faeces. This procedure should be supplemented by repeated enemata, and further manual evacuations as required.

TUBES AND DRAINS IN THE ABDOMINAL CAVITY

Drains and tubes placed in the abdominal cavity are often a source of concern to a surgical houseman. He may be unsure of the purpose of the drain, the location of the drain within the abdominal cavity, and when and how it should be removed. These questions can be solved either by being present at the operation itself or by questioning the surgeon involved. In general abdominal drains are used either to remove fluid already present within the abdominal cavity such as pus, bile, faeces or blood, or to remove such fluids should a bowel anastomosis break down or biliary or pancreatic leakage occur. The character of the fluid should therefore be carefully noted for the presence of pus, blood, bile, small bowel content, pancreatic secretions or ascitic fluid. Specimens should be sent to the laboratory where necessary to confirm the nature of these secretions. An assessment of the 24 hour volume of the secretions should be made. It is difficult to give general rules on the removal of such drains since they will depend on the nature of the secretions, and on the requirements of the surgeon involved. Make sure that you, and the nursing staff, are familiar with these requirements otherwise mistakes will be made. The removal of abdominal drains is performed by gradually shortening the drain 2 to 5 cm daily until removal is completed.

A special case of intra-abdominal drain is the T-tube used in biliary surgery. The T-tube is inserted into the common bile duct and the long end brought out through the skin through a separate stab incision. Bile is drained into a bag for five to seven days, when the T-tube is clamped. If free drainage of bile into the duodenum does not occur then clamping of the T-tube will result in pain and tenderness in the right hypochondrium and the clamp should be removed immediately. A T-tube cholangiogram to check for residual stones and obstruction should always be performed before removal of the tube. This should be done in stages over a period of three to four days. There is usually a small leakage of bile from the drain site but if the common bile duct is not obstructed it ceases very rapidly.

OESOPHAGOSCOPY, FIBROSCOPY AND GASTROSCOPY

For diagnostic purposes flexible fibroptic instruments with side or end viewing are used. For removal of foreign bodies from the oesophagus, a rigid instrument is more useful.

For these procedures the patient is prepared by fasting overnight. One hour beforehand pre-medication using Omnopon, morphine or diazepam is given (*see* Chapter 2). At the same time the patient is given a local anaesthetic lozenge (amethocaine hydrochloride lozenge; 60 mg) to suck, and a second lozenge is given half an hour before the procedure.

The patient lies on his right side and is blindfolded. The instrument is then gently introduced through the mouth and into the stomach or oesophagus. At the end of the procedure the patient is warned not to take food or fluid for three hours, until the local anaesthetic has worn off. If oesophagoscopy and biopsy have been performed the patient is admitted and observed overnight and water only given in case perforation of the oesophagus has occurred. A chest X-ray should be carried out before discharging the patient.

PROCTOSCOPY, SIGMOIDOSCOPY AND COLONOSCOPY

Preparation of the bowel prior to these procedures is important since the success of the examination will be determined by the visibility. It is usual for the patient to be given a soap and water enema in the hour before the procedure and in most cases this gives a satisfactory view. For the outpatient, a disposable enema is given to the patient, along with careful instructions as to the mode of administration. The enema itself is administered a few hours before the examination. If the examination is to be carried out in the afternoon a light breakfast but no lunch can be taken. Colonoscopy using the flexible fibroptic colonoscope requires much more careful preparation with repeated enemas.

Proctoscopy requires little preparation of the patient and should be carried out as a routine part of the physical examination. It is preceded by a careful rectal examination. The well lubricated proctoscope with obturator is then introduced into the anal canal and lower rectum. The obturator is removed and observations as to the character of the rectal mucosa and anal canal are made.

Sigmoidoscopy is usually carried out with the patient in the left lateral position. It is important that the patient comes close to the edge of the table with the knees drawn up to the chest. A general anaesthetic is not usually employed since the use of excessive force, which would be painful in the non-anaesthetised patient and result in the termination of the sigmoidoscopy, may cause perforation of the large bowel if the patient is anaesthetised. It is of course very important to explain the procedure fully to the patient before commencing and during the course of the manoeuvre to let him know what is happening.

Before sigmoidoscopy is carried out a rectal examination should be performed so that any abnormality of the anus or lower rectum can be noted. It will also ensure that local painful conditions of the anus are detected before insertion of the sigmoidoscope. The well lubricated instrument with obturator is then inserted with gentle rotary movements to overcome the tone of the anal sphincter. The obturator is then removed and under direct vision the sigmoidoscope is passed gently upwards, the bowel being distended with air. At the recto-sigmoid junction special care is taken since undue force may cause perforation of the colon. If at any stage the patient complains of severe pain, or becomes restless and agitated the sigmoidoscope should be withdrawn immediately under direct vision and the procedure abandoned.

During the procedure observations are made of the anus, the surrounding skin, anal tone, the presence of haemorrhoids, or other abnormalities. As the sigmoidoscope is inserted, note is made of the character of the mucosa, the presence of blood or pus, the presence of tumours, ulcers or polyps. At each stage the level in centimetres from the anal margin is measured as is the maximum distance of insertion of the sigmoidoscope. Biopsies are taken as required.

Insertion of the colonoscope is similar to that described under sigmoidoscopy, and a specially made split sigmoidoscope may be used to facilitate its entry. The advancing end of the instrument can be manipulated by a control mounted at the other end and by this means the colonoscope can negotiate the recto-sigmoid junction and reach the descending colon.

LIVER BIOPSY (Figure 27)

Biopsy of the liver can be carried out either at operation or with a needle, under local or general anaesthesia. The Vim-Silverman or Menghini needle or one of their modifications is used. To screen for a coagulation defect the patient should have a normal prothrombin time, platelet count and bleeding time. The patient is started on vitamin K before the procedure is carried out, and one litre of blood is cross-matched.

The needle is usually inserted intercostally at the point of maximum liver dullness in the anterior axillary line, the patient lying obliquely on his left side. If the liver is clearly palpable below the costal margin, a biopsy may be taken from this site. After the procedure the patient is closely observed overnight in case bleeding or biliary leakage occur. An hourly pulse and blood pressure are recorded.

SMALL BOWEL BIOPSY (Figure 27)

Since this procedure is often carried out on patients with malabsorption or anaemia, the haematological status of the

LIVER AND SMALL BOWEL BIOPSY

LIVER BIOPSY

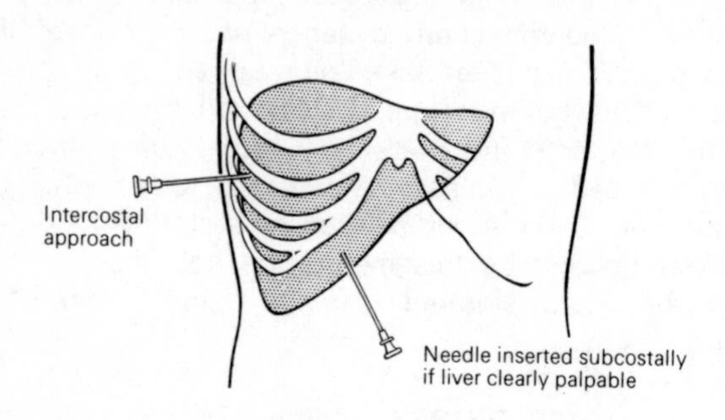

SCHEMATIC REPRESENTATION OF SMALL BOWEL BIOPSY

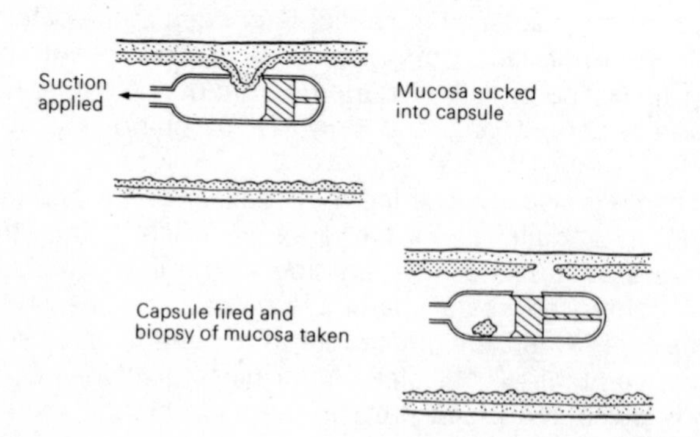

Figure 27

patient, and in particular the coagulation mechanisms and platelet count, should be checked prior to the test. The small bowel biopsy capsule (the Crosby-Kugler capsule or modification), ready loaded and attached to fine bore tubing is swallowed by the patient, and the end of the tubing securely fixed to the face. Over the next 12 hours the patient is allowed to eat and drink normally as the tube and capsule gradually pass down through the stomach into the small bowel. Before taking the biopsy the position of the tube is checked radiologically in case the capsule has not negotiated the pylorus. The X-ray will also give some idea as to the site of the capsule. With a 10 ml syringe, suction is applied, the small bowel mucosa being sucked into the capsule. The mucosa is then cut by firing the capsule and the tube, with biopsy, removed by gentle traction.

10. ABDOMINAL PARACENTESIS

The removal of fluid from the abdominal cavity is a useful diagnostic and therapeutic technique. Two methods are available; the first uses the trocar and cannula, and the second, the newer plastic catheters (Figure 28).

1. Insertion of trocar and cannula

Before starting make sure that all equipment is available. You will require a trocar and cannula, local anaesthetic, swabs, antiseptic solutions and a receptacle to collect the fluid. A knife handle and blade will also be required. Many hospitals have a pack containing equipment for abdominal paracentesis. Make sure that you know what material is available and that the trocar and cannula fit correctly. Check that the drainage tubing fits the end of the cannula before starting. Note that ordinary drip set tubing may fit the cannula and this is not only easy to obtain but has a regulator attached making adjustment of the drainage rate a simple matter.

Two sites can be used for abdominal paracentesis. The first is mid-way between the symphysis pubis and the umbilicus in the mid-line. The major danger here is that the bladder may be damaged so always make sure the bladder is empty. The alternative site is in the right or left iliac fossa between the umbilicus and anterior superior iliac spine. Note the usual position of the inferior epigastric artery (Figure 28).

After infiltrating the skin with local anaesthetic make a small nick in the skin with a knife and insert the trocar and cannula through skin, muscle and peritoneum. When the peritoneum has been punctured, there is a definite feeling of giving way. Remember that the skin and subcutaneous tissue in a patient with gross ascites may be very thin and only gentle pressure with the trocar will be required. Remove the trocar and connect the cannula to a bag for the collection of ascitic fluid. A few swabs are placed round the cannula which is then taped in position.

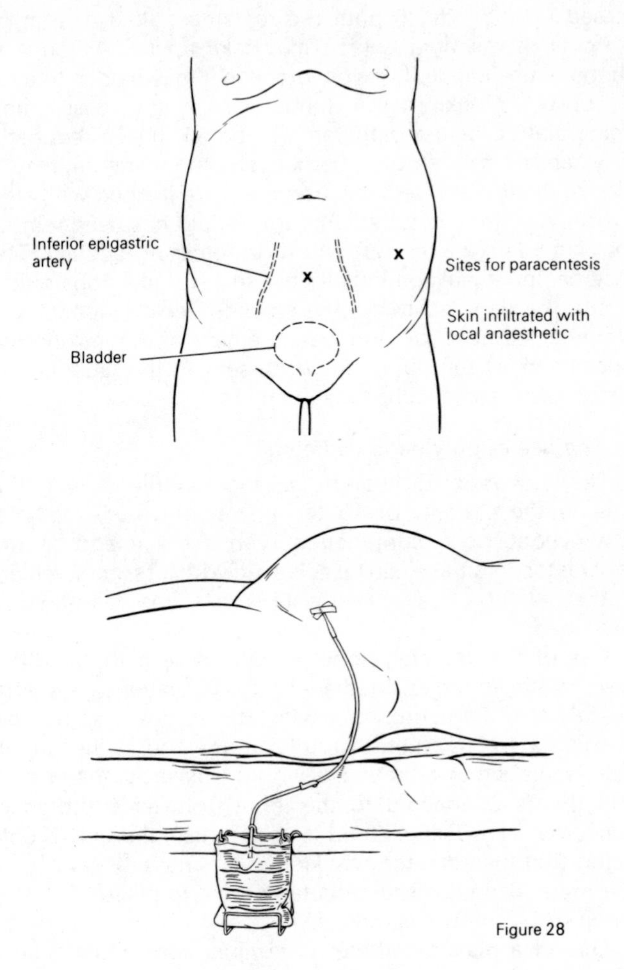
ABDOMINAL PARACENTESIS
Inferior epigastric artery
x
x
Sites for paracentesis
Skin infiltrated with local anaesthetic
Bladder

Figure 28

In the patient with gross ascites rapid decompression can be dangerous and some form of spring clip should be used to regulate the flow of fluid. As the abdomen becomes less tense the rate of flow will fall. If the cannula has been inserted into one of the iliac fossae the patient should be turned on his side to pool the remaining fluid. During the removal of the fluid, which may take up to 24 hours, the cannula may block. If this occurs then it may be due to a loop of bowel blocking the lumen, in which case simple manipulation of the catheter may be all that is required to re-establish free flow. Alternatively the cannula may be blocked with fibrin and may require to be flushed with sterile saline. When the required amount of fluid has been removed the cannula is pulled out and a dry dressing applied. There may be some leakage initially but this usually stops quickly. If not, then an ileostomy bag placed over the puncture site will enable collection and measurement of the leaking fluid. Specimens of the fluid should be sent to the laboratory for histological and biochemical analysis.

2. The use of polythene catheters

The conventional metal trocar and cannula is uncomfortable to the patient. Using the newer polythene catheters, either alone or in conjunction with a trocar and cannula, satisfactory drainage can be achieved with less inconvenience to the patient. Local anaesthesia is performed as previously described.

Use of the catheter alone. A wide bore catheter (30 cm long) with attached needle (12 to 16 gauge), is inserted directly into the peritoneal cavity. Before doing so however, it is useful to cut additional holes in the end of the catheter. The needle is then removed leaving the plastic catheter *in situ,* and this is connected to the length of sterile tubing and collection bag. This method is easy to use, the only problem being that the catheter may kink and block more easily than the metal cannula. The catheter is held in place by a single stitch or by the use of adhesive tape.

Use of a plastic catheter in conjunction with trocar and cannula. After insertion of the trocar and cannula as described above, a polythene catheter (30 cm long) of suitable thickness (approx. 14 gauge) is inserted through the cannula which is then withdrawn. Make sure however that the catheter fits before starting the procedure.

Diagnostic paracentesis of the peritoneal cavity

This procedure has been recommended as a diagnostic tool in cases of trauma to the abdomen, or in the undiagnosed acute abdomen. A 2.5 ml syringe, local anaesthetic and a 12 to 14 gauge needle are required. Alternatively a spinal puncture needle may be used. After cleaning the skin and infiltrating with local anaesthetic the needle is inserted through the abdominal wall into the peritoneal cavity and gently moved about while the syringe is intermittently sucked. The needle is inserted either at the point of maximum tenderness or separately in all four quadrants of the abdomen. The latter method reduces the number of false negative results. The tap is regarded as significant if more than 0.5 ml are obtained. After inspection of the sample for blood, bile or turbidity it is sent for appropriate laboratory examination.

11. THE MAINTENANCE OF AN ADEQUATE AIRWAY

In the unconscious patient, or in the patient with acute respiratory obstruction or respiratory arrest, the establishment of an adequate airway is a life-saving procedure.

In the unconscious patient, without respiratory problems, the simplest way to maintain a clear airway is by correct positioning. The patient should be placed in the prone, or semi-prone position, with the foot of the bed elevated (Figure 29). In this position the tongue falls forwards and any saliva, blood or gastric content will dribble out rather than be aspirated into the trachea. An airway placed over the tongue will prevent it falling backwards, occluding the air passages. If, for any reason, the unconscious patient is in the supine position, the angle of jaw should be pulled upwards (Figure 29) to prevent the tongue from blocking the airway. Frequent suction of the mouth and pharynx may be necessary to remove secretions. These simple measures should prevent most of the respiratory complications in the unconscious patient.

If respiratory difficulty occurs in the conscious or unconscious patient other procedures such as laryngoscopy, bronchoscopy, endotracheal intubation, laryngostomy or tracheostomy may be required.

LARYNGOSCOPY

In any patient with stridor, laryngoscopy should be carried out as an emergency procedure. Stridor may be due to paralysis of the vocal chords or to a plug of mucus in the larynx. The laryngoscope is inserted, the operator standing behind the patient who lies supine. As a first step, since the patient is usually fully conscious, the fauces and pharynx are sprayed with a local anaesthetic solution (such as 4 per cent lignocaine) as described in detail under bronchoscopy. The vocal chords are visualised and movement of them noted (Figure 31). Any pus or mucus is sucked from the larynx. Following this procedure, if local anaesthesia has been used,

POSITIONING OF THE UNCONSCIOUS PATIENT

JAW HELD UPWARDS TO PREVENT
TONGUE FROM FALLING BACK

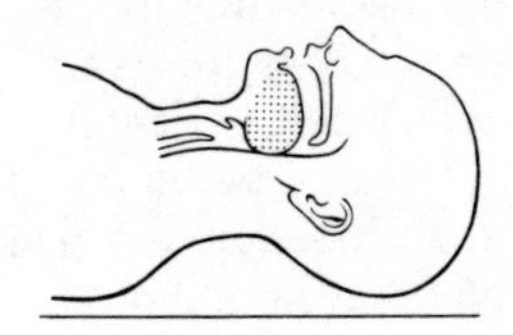

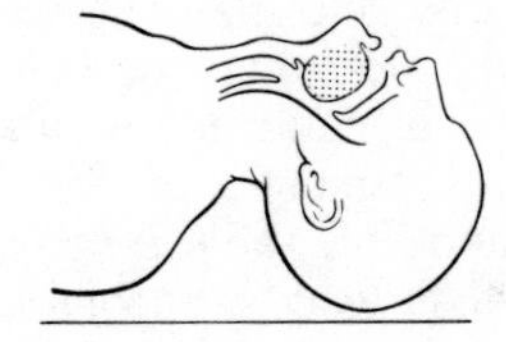

NURSING POSITION FOR THE
UNCONSCIOUS PATIENT

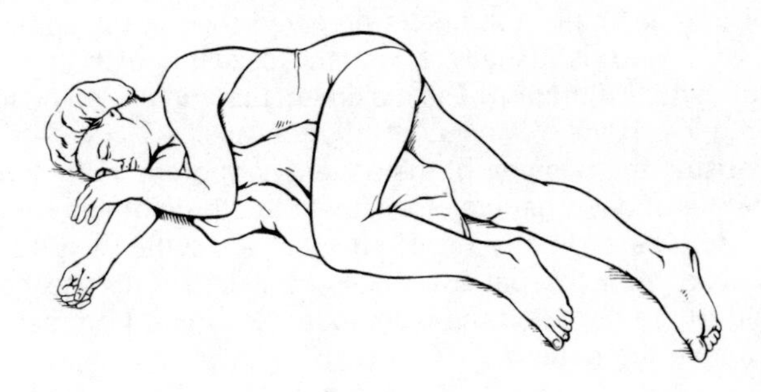

Figure 29

the patient should take nothing orally for three hours in case aspiration of the fluid into the trachea occurs.

BRONCHOSCOPY (Figure 30)

In the emergency situation for the removal of bronchial or tracheal secretions this procedure may be performed in the very ill patient under local anaesthetic. Usually however, it is carried out as an elective procedure under a general anaesthetic, and the patient is prepared for this in the usual way. The procedure may be carried out in the ward or in theatre. Pre-medication is not essential but is useful if time permits. Diagnostic bronchoscopy is the province of the expert and only the essentials of the procedure are given to enable emergency bronchial suction to be carried out.

Before starting check the bronchoscope and its lighting. Efficient and powerful suction will be required as will biopsy forceps and a trap for the collection of sputum. To carry out the procedure under local anaesthesia the throat and larynx are sprayed under direct vision using a laryngoscope with a local anaesthetic such as 4 per cent lignocaine. This strength of local anaesthetic solution is prepared for surface application only and is usually coloured to distinguish it from solutions for infiltration. The maximum recommended dose is 100 mg, i.e. 10 ml of 4 per cent solution.

As usual the position of the patient is of great importance. In theatre under a general anaesthetic the patient lies supine with shoulders slightly raised. If local anaesthesia is to be employed then the patient is sat up in bed with the head turned to the right and the technique performed from behind and above the patient.

Method of insertion of bronchoscope under local anaesthesia

The patient's eyes are first covered with a towel and the upper jaw pulled upwards by swabs held under the upper teeth. The tongue is pulled forwards and the bronchoscope inserted, the epiglottis being pushed anteriorly. At first the bronchoscope is inserted so that the advancing edge is

BRONCHOSCOPY

POSITIONING FOR BRONCHOSCOPY IN THE POST-OPERATIVE PATIENT

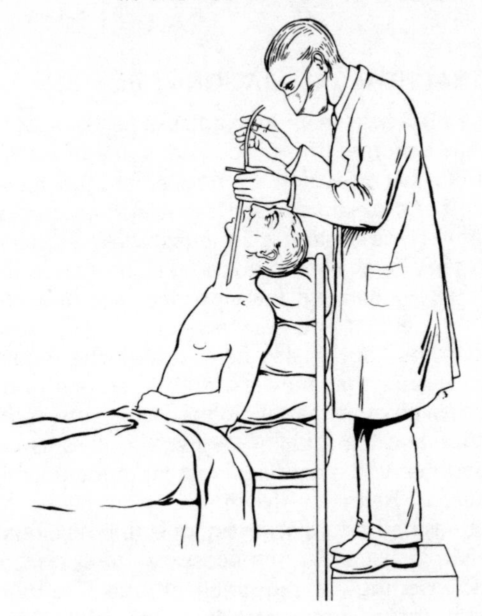

POSITION FOR DIAGNOSTIC BRONCHOSCOPY

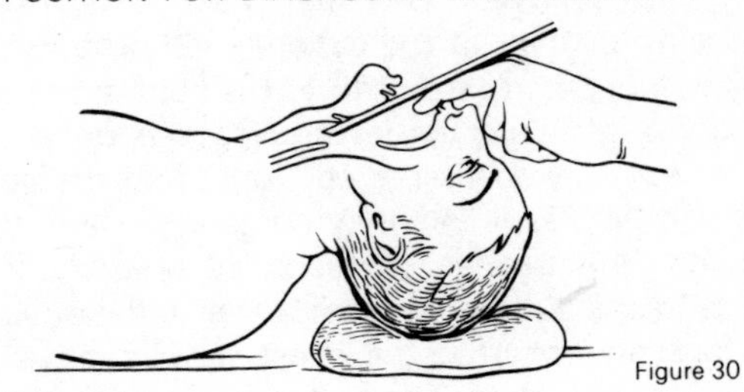

Figure 30

anterior. When the vocal cords are visualised it is rotated at right angles so that the advancing edge is now in line with the vocal cords. The bronchoscope is inserted through the cords and the carina visualised. Both sides of the bronchial tree are examined and suction or biopsy carried out as required.

ENDOTRACHEAL INTUBATION (Figure 31)

In patients with acute respiratory disorders or in whom cardiac arrest has occurred, this procedure is one of the most important and life-saving which the houseman may have to perform. With other procedures such as intravenous therapy, blood sampling or the insertion of chest drains, there is usually time to seek help. With endotracheal intubation there is usually not. It is imperative therefore that the houseman knows where the nearest endotracheal tube, laryngoscope, and inflation bag are kept. These items should be regularly checked to make sure that they are still in working order, have not been moved, and that all connections between the endotracheal tube and the inflation bag still fit. It is usual to keep such apparatus with a cardiac arrest kit in a convenient place in the ward or Recovery Room.

If the patient has had a cardiac arrest, or is unconscious for other reasons, it is usually not necessary to use muscle relaxants before inserting the endotracheal tube. The patient lies supine with the operator standing behind his head. Dentures are removed. The laryngoscope is inserted, the tongue being pushed to the patient's left. The endotracheal tube ready lubricated (size 8 to 11) is held in the right hand and with the left hand the laryngoscope is pulled upwards. This manoeuvre exposes the epiglottis and the vocal cords should then be visible. As they come into view, the tube is slipped into the trachea. As soon as possible the cuff is inflated and the tube connected to an inflation bag. If the tube is properly inserted the chest should move uniformly with manual ventilation. The cuff makes sure that the trachea is air-tight and prevents aspiration of gastric contents or saliva into the bronchi. For females a number 8 or 9 tube is usually

ENDOTRACHEAL INTUBATION

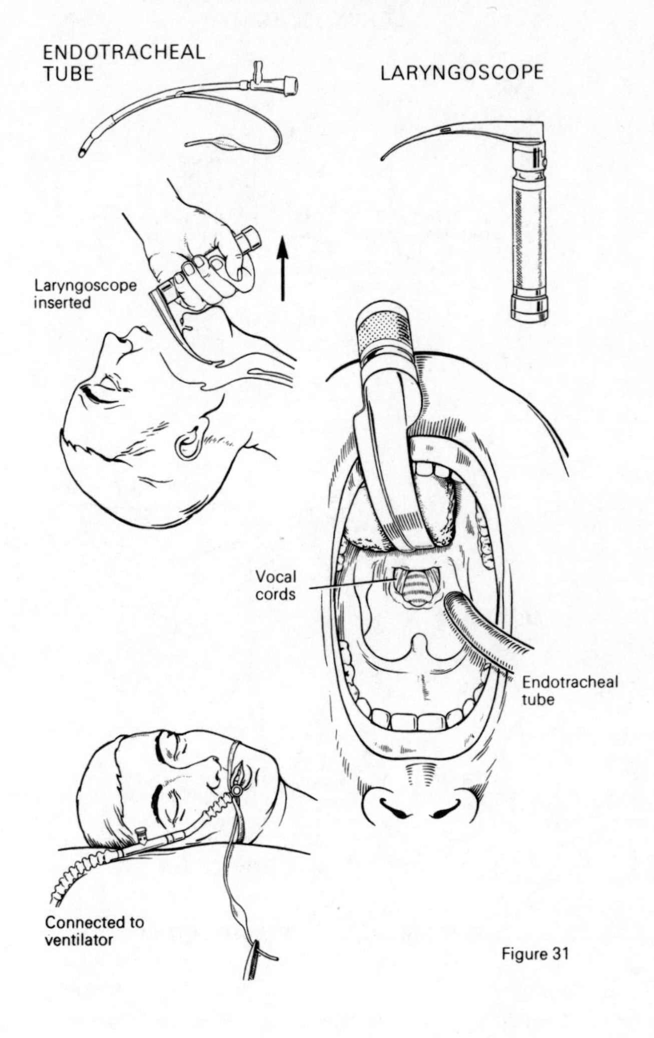

Figure 31

LARYNGOSTOMY

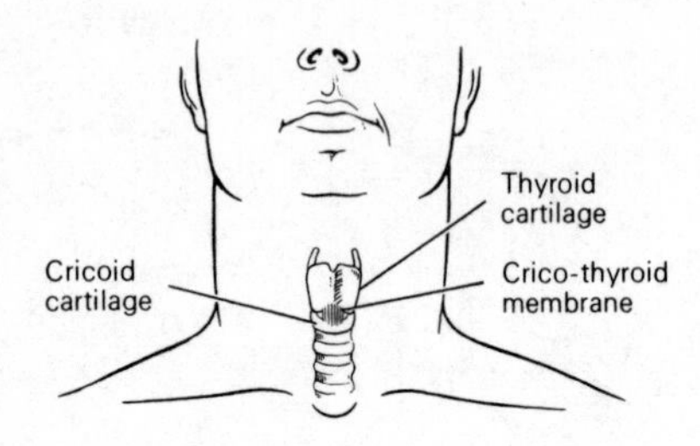

METHOD 1

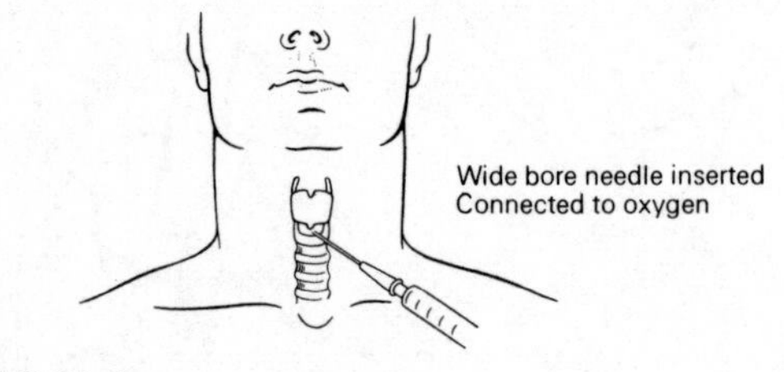

METHOD 2

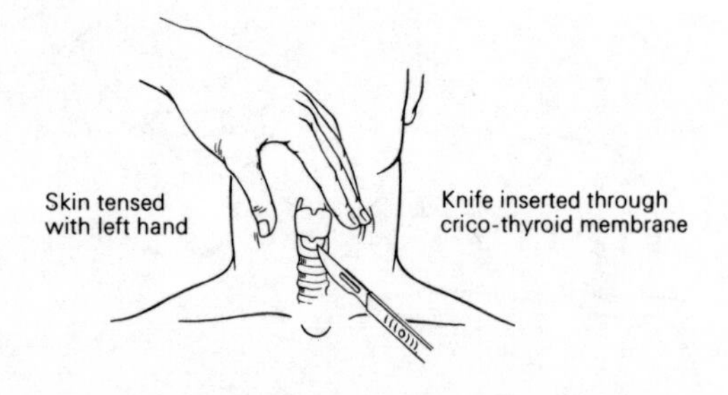

THEN PROCEED TO TRACHEOSTOMY

Figure 32

adequate; for males sizes 9 to 11 are suitable depending on the build of the patient. Both rubber and synthetic plastic tubes are available but the latter are better for long-term use.

If the endotracheal tube is to be inserted and the patient requires relaxation, there is usually time to contact an anaesthetist. He will usually give 50 to 100 mg of suxamethonium chloride following 5 to 6 ml of 2.5 per cent thiopentone or other short acting anaesthetic, or induce anaesthesia with nitrous oxide or halothane. When relaxation is complete, usually within a few seconds, the tube is rapidly inserted and the patient ventilated. By resorting to the use of muscle relaxants an irreversible step has been taken in that skilled assistance must be available in case it is not possible to pass the endotracheal tube. The houseman should therefore not carry out this procedure on his own. The care of the patient with an endotracheal tube will be discussed in the section on tracheostomy.

Description of the technique is no substitute for practice, and this can be done most easily during the induction of anaesthesia. All medical students and housemen should have the opportunity to pass an endotracheal tube under supervision.

It is usually recommended that an endotracheal tube should not remain in position for more than 48 hours. With the newer PVC tubes this period may be extended, but tracheostomy should be considered if long term intubation is required.

TRACHEOSTOMY AND LARYNGOSTOMY

Tracheostomy should normally be performed in the operating theatre or intensive care unit with a general anaesthetic. It should be regarded as an elective procedure and an endotracheal tube should be in position before starting. Under circumstances of acute laryngeal obstruction or respiratory failure where an endotracheal tube cannot be passed, tracheostomy should not be attempted as an emergency procedure but laryngostomy performed.

Laryngostomy (Figure 32)

As indicated this procedure should be undertaken in circumstances of acute laryngeal obstruction, where an endotracheal tube cannot be passed. It has complications, such as stenosis and inflammation of the larynx, but if the technique is used as a temporary life-saving procedure then these risks may be justifiable. Certainly it is better than an emergency tracheostomy in inexperienced hands. Several methods are available. Perhaps the simplest is to thrust a wide bore needle 12 to 14 gauge, through the space between the thyroid cartilage and the cricoid cartilage, the cricothyroid membrane. This needle is then connected to a cylinder of oxygen. Alternatively, with the thumb and index finger of the left hand tensing the skin, an incision is made over the cricothyroid membrane which is then separately incised. This procedure is very rapid and by simply turning the handle of the scalpel in the wound, an adequate airway can be established until a laryngostomy tube is available.

It is emphasised that this is a temporary procedure which must be followed as soon as possible, by formal tracheostomy and closure of the wound.

Elective tracheostomy (Figures 33, 34)

This is usually performed under general anaesthesia but local anaesthesia may be necessary in some cases. An endotracheal tube should be in place. Before anaesthetisation, if the patient is conscious, he should be fully informed of the procedure and in particular warned that he will be unable to speak after the procedure is completed. Full sterile precautions are used and if possible the procedure is carried out in the operating theatre. Before starting make sure that there is adequate lighting and that a variety of sizes of tracheostomy tubes are available. Tracheostomy tubes may be of silver or polyvinyl chloride (PVC). The PVC tubes are the least irritant and are available in sizes 24 to 42 French gauge. For the average male, sizes 36 to 39 should be suitable and for females sizes 33 to 36. These tubes are cuffed and some tubes have double cuffs to minimise tracheal trauma.

TRACHEOSTOMY I

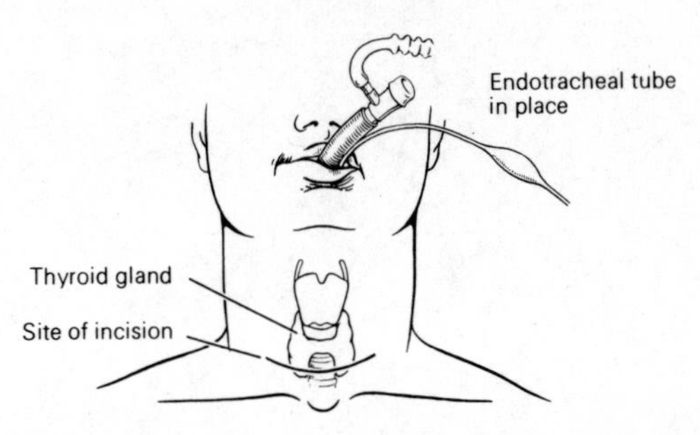

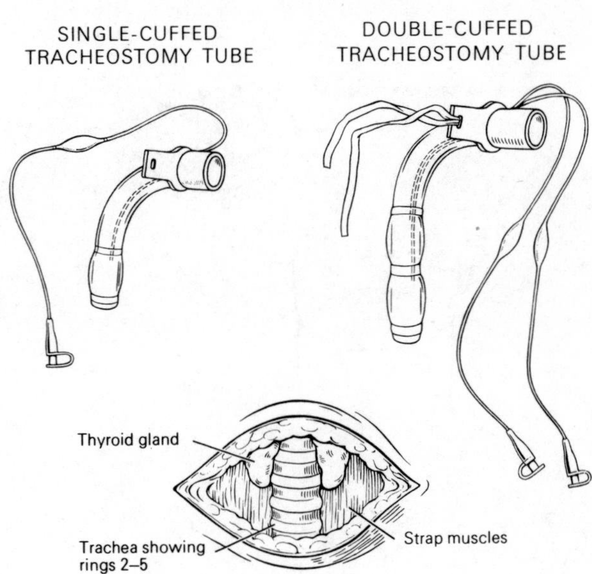

Figure 33

TRACHEOSTOMY II

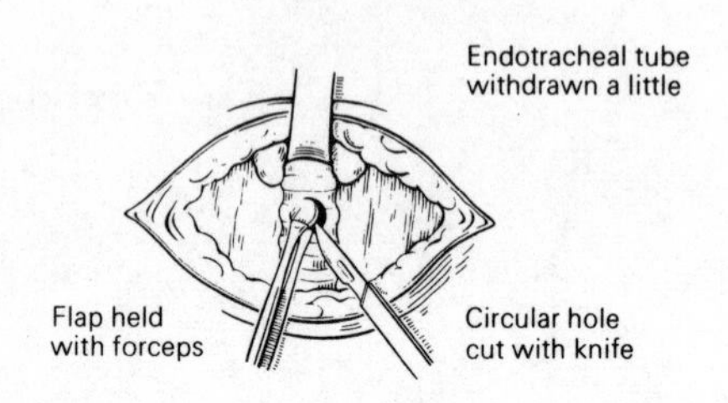

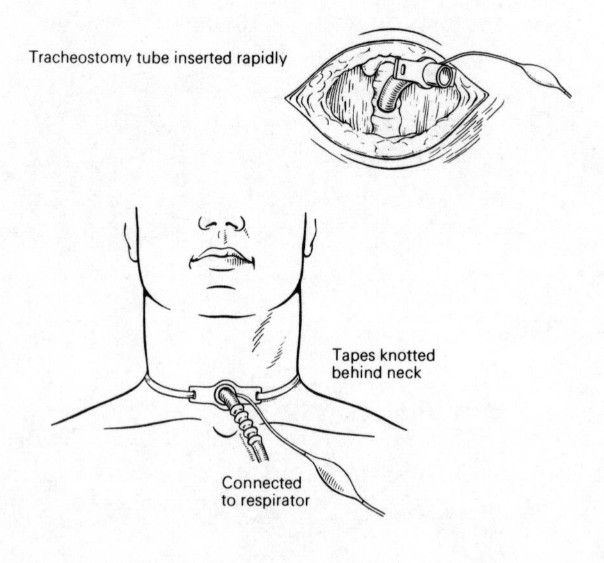

Figure 34

A transverse incision is made in the skin of the neck 4 to 5 cm long midway between the cricoid cartilage and the suprasternal notch and the tissues divided in this line down to the deep fascia. The strap muscles are then cut vertically in the midline and the trachea exposed. All bleeding must be stopped before further incisions are made. The cricoid cartilage is palpated as is the first tracheal ring. It is imperative that the first tracheal cartilage is *not* incised or stenosis will occur. It may not be possible to see tracheal rings 2 to 5 because of overlying thyroid tissue and if this is the case the thyroid isthmus is retracted or divided. Artery forceps are used to clamp either side of the thyroid, which is then divided between them exposing the trachea. At this point it is worthwhile comparing the size of the trachea with the proposed tracheostomy tube. The endotracheal tube is withdrawn a little prior to opening the trachea since if difficulties arise the tube may be replaced rapidly.

Several methods may be used to open the trachea but the simplest is to cut out a circular hole. The incision is commenced and artery forceps or tissue forceps placed on the cartilage so that there is no chance of the portion removed falling into the trachea. The forceps having been applied, the incision is completed and the circle of trachea removed. As rapidly as possible the tracheostomy tube is inserted. It may be useful at this point to use tracheal dilators. Remember, if the patient is anaesthetised and paralysed there will be no oxygen reaching the lungs during this time and intubation must therefore be carried out with urgency.

The second method of opening the trachea is to use a ∩-shaped incision, the flap being turned down and sutured to the lower edge of the skin with catgut. This method makes it easier to change the tube in the early stages after tracheostomy. In either event the tracheostomy tube is quickly connected to the anaesthetic machine so that oxygenation and anaesthesia may be recommenced. The cuff of the tracheostomy tube is then inflated and the ends of the wound loosely sutured. The tapes of the tracheostomy tube are then securely knotted together at the back of the neck. It is important that the ends are knotted since it is easy for them to be loosened in mistake for the patient's gown. The tracheostomy, tube itself may then be sutured to the skin with two stitches. Swabs are placed under the tracheostomy tube at either end.

Care of the tracheostomy. The indications for tracheostomy usually mean that the patient, at least initially, will require frequent tracheal toilet to remove retained secretions. This should be done as a sterile procedure, masks and gloves being worn. A strong suction machine, sterile suction catheters and saline are required. Using forceps the catheter is inserted into the trachea and suction is applied only as the tube is removed. The catheter is inserted into one main bronchus then the other. Depending on the clinical state of the patient, suction is repeated as often as required, which may be every 15 to 30 minutes initially.

Since the cuff of the tracheostomy tube will cause pressure on the trachea it is usual to deflate it for a period of five minutes every two hours. Since deflation often induces coughing the trachea should be sucked out prior to deflation, after deflation, and after re-inflation.

Changing the tracheostomy tube. Once again full sterile precautions should be undertaken. The equipment for tracheal suction should be available as should a tracheostomy tube of the same size together with one of a smaller size. The tapes securing the tracheostomy tube are cut and the dressings taken down. The tracheostomy is then sucked out, the cuff deflated, and suction repeated. The tube is then gently removed and the new one inserted as soon as possible. Suction is then repeated. A smaller tube must always be available in case the tube cannot be re-inserted; this cannot be over-emphasised since fatalities have been recorded due to failure to re-intubate the patient.

The conscious patient and the tracheostomy tube. Some conscious patients with a tracheostomy tube or endotracheal tube rapidly adapt to the situation even if assisted ventilation is being used. Reassurance and explanation may be all that is required. With other patients however, the presence of the tube in the trachea together with associated injuries make them restless and sedation will be required. When sedation only is required phenoperidine 2 mg intravenously may be sufficient, the dose being repeated as required, unless the blood pressure is reduced by the drug. Phenoperidine may also be used in conjunction with droperidol, 5 to 10 mg being given intravenously if more sedation is required. Diazepam 2 to 10 mg may be used if sedation only is necessary. If relaxation of a patient being ventilated is necessary then a muscle relaxant such as pancuronium, 4 mg intravenously may be administered.

Removal of the tracheostomy tube. It is necessary to do this at the earliest possible date compatible with the clinical state of the patient to minimise the dangers of long-term tracheostomy. With this procedure, as with changing of the tracheostomy tube, it is imperative that a second, smaller tube is available in case laryngeal obstruction, or obstruction at the stoma occurs. Before removing the tube the cuff is deflated for two to three days and the stoma covered with a swab. If the trachea and upper air passages are patent then the patient should be able to speak and breathe normally. This will however not exclude an area of granulation tissue above the tube which on its removal will block the lumen. It is therefore recommended that before removal of the tube, a lateral soft tissue X-ray of the neck is performed to exclude obstruction higher up in the trachea. Following removal the patient must be closely observed over the next few hours for increasing respiratory difficulty, cyanosis or stridor. If any of these occur the patient should be re-intubated immediately. After successful removal of the tube it is not usually necessary to insert stitches into the wound.

12. DRAINAGE OF THE PLEURAL CAVITY

INSERTION OF INTERCOSTAL DRAIN FOR PNEUMOTHORAX (Figure 35)

Emergency drainage

In the emergency situation with a tension pneumothorax causing severe respiratory embarrassment there may be no time to insert a formal intercostal drain. In this case a wide bore needle or intravenous cannula should be thrust directly through the chest wall in the second interspace just outside the mid-clavicular line. Suction can then be applied to the needle. A definitive intercostal drain can then be inserted when the equipment is available.

Formal drainage using trocar and cannula

Before commencing it is important to check both by clinical examination and by examining the chest X-ray of the patient that the correct side is being drained. Explain the procedure to the patient. Check that the trocar and cannula fit, and ensure that the malecot catheter plus introducer will go through the cannula. Have a heavy clamp ready, and the apparatus for closed water-seal drainage available. The procedure is carried out with full aseptic precautions. A number 26 to 28 French Gauge malecot catheter is usually adequate.

Local anaesthetic is infiltrated under the skin of the chest wall in the 2nd intercostal space just outside the mid-clavicular line. The muscle layers and pleura are then anaesthetised using a wider bore and longer needle. A small transverse incision is made in the skin with a knife and the trocar and cannula pushed through into the pleural cavity. This procedure often takes a considerable amount of pressure and this should be explained to the patient. There is an obvious decrease in resistance as the pleura is penetrated. It is important to note that the trocar should be kept as close as possible to the lower rib to avoid damage to the intercostal vessels. The trocar is removed and a finger or thumb placed over the opening of the cannula. The catheter and introducer

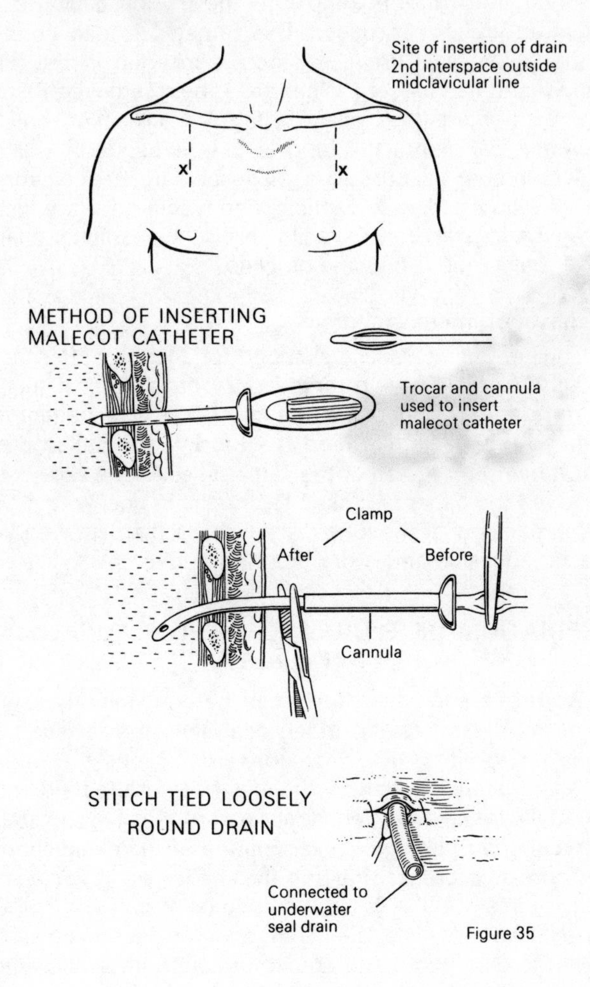
INSERTION OF INTERCOSTAL DRAIN FOR PNEUMOTHORAX
Site of insertion of drain
2nd interspace outside
midclavicular line
x
x
METHOD OF INSERTING
MALECOT CATHETER
Trocar and cannula
used to insert
malecot catheter
Clamp
After
Before
Cannula
STITCH TIED LOOSELY
ROUND DRAIN
Connected to
underwater
seal drain

Figure 35

are then quickly inserted and the cannula and introducer removed. During this manoeuvre it is important that, as the introducer is removed, the catheter is clamped firmly. This, first of all, prevents air escaping and secondly, prevents the catheter from disappearing into the pleural cavity, a complication which can occur. The catheter is then connected to the water-seal drain. A stitch is inserted in the manner shown and tied loosely. When the tube is removed this stitch can be tightened. A chest X-ray is then taken and films repeated daily until the lung is fully expanded.

A commercially produced, disposable trocar and cannula is now available (Argyle) which is convenient for the insertion of an intercostal drain. A facility is also available for changing the tube should it become blocked.

Removal of intercostal drain

The catheter is usually clamped for 24 hours after the lung is fully expanded, then removed 24 hours later if there has been no recurrence of the pneumothorax. The patient is first sedated with pethidine and the tube gently pulled out, the stitch being tightened at the same time. As the tube is being removed the patient is asked to breathe in deeply to maintain full expansion of the lungs. The area is then sprayed with a plastic adhesive and a dry dressing applied.

ASPIRATION OF FLUID FROM THE PLEURAL CAVITY (Figure 36)

Both pus and other fluids can be conveniently aspirated from the pleural cavity under local anaesthesia. The patient is asked to sit up and lean forwards. A chest X-ray, both P-A and lateral, will show the exact site of the fluid and this is usually in the most dependent part of the chest, posteriorly. Clinical and radiological examination of the chest should be performed before starting and the site for aspiration selected. This is usually in the 8th or 9th intercostal space in the posterior axillary line. A needle inserted lower than this may penetrate the diaphragm and spread infection into the peritoneal cavity.

ASPIRATION OF PLEURAL FLUID—INSERTION OF INTERCOSTAL DRAIN

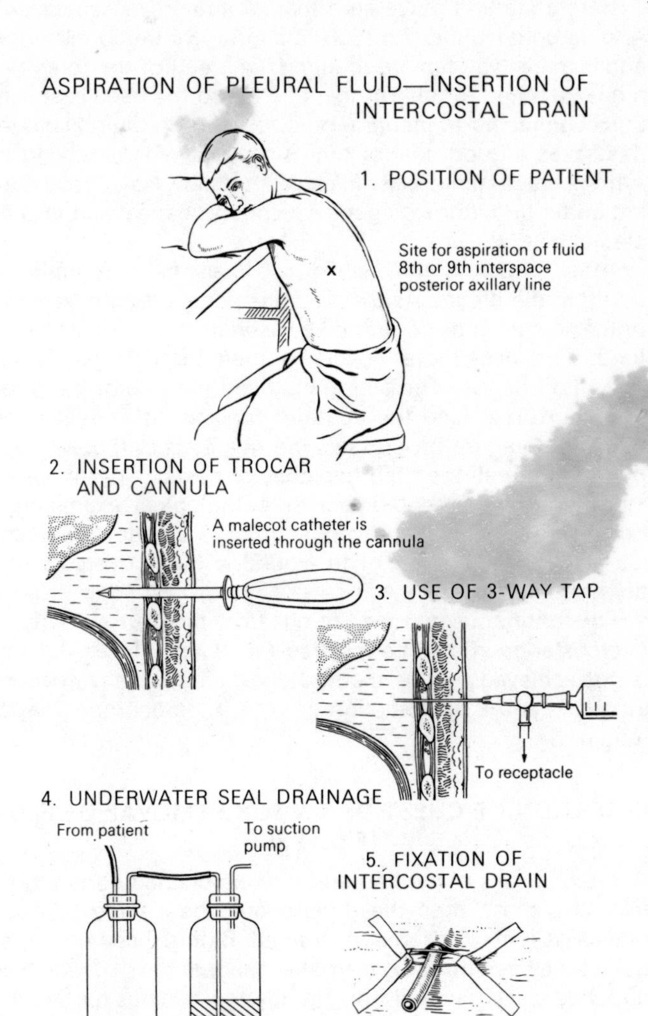

Figure 36

Before starting make sure that all equipment is available. A wide bore needle, 7.5 to 10 cm long, with a 50 ml syringe and a three-way tap are required. One end of the three-way tap is attached to the syringe, another to the needle, and the third connected to sterile tubing to drain the fluid aspirated, this saves a good deal of time since it avoids removing the syringe each time it is filled with fluid. Have ready any antibiotic or cytotoxic agent which is to be instilled into the pleural cavity.

After preparing the skin, local anaesthetic is infiltrated down to the pleura. As the pleura is penetrated the accuracy of the siting can be confirmed by aspirating a small amount of fluid. The wide bore needle is then inserted gently and aspiration begun. The syringe is filled with fluid, the three-way tap turned and the contents flushed into a receptacle. As the procedure progresses, the needle is withdrawn little by little until all the fluid has been removed. Specimens are then sent for bacteriological or pathological examination. Before the needle is removed, antibiotics or cytotoxic agents are instilled as required. The wound is then covered with a dry dressing.

For continuous drainage of pus from the pleural cavity, an intercostal drain may be inserted (see later). If free drainage is not achieved by this method, the fluid may have become loculated and a rib resection or even a thoracotomy may be required.

INSERTION OF CHEST DRAIN FOR REMOVAL OF FLUID (Figure 36)

If blood, pus or pleural fluid is to be drained continuously from the chest, then the drain should be a wide bore one otherwise it may become obstructed. Before inserting a chest drain for a haemothorax, the patient should have blood cross-matched, a 'drip' should be set up, and transfusion begun if necessary since 1 to 2 litres of blood can rapidly collect in this situation.

The procedure is carried out under local anaesthesia. The patient sits up, leaning forwards with arms resting on pillows. Before starting check that a wide bore tube is available, and that artery forceps and clamps are ready. A water-seal drain is set up and all connections checked to make sure that they fit and are air-tight. The skin is then cleaned with antiseptic solution and the skin, muscle and pleura infiltrated with local anaesthetic. The usual site for insertion of the drain is in the 8th or 9th intercostal spaces in the posterior axillary line. If a large malecot catheter is available then it may be inserted using a trocar and cannula. After infiltrating with local anaesthetic a small skin incision is made. Using a trocar and cannula the site of insertion should be no lower than the 9th interspace because of the danger of damaging subdiaphragmatic viscera. By the same token, the trocar should be directed towards the opposite axilla to avoid going through the diaphragm. The malecot catheter is inserted as described under pneumothorax.

If a wide bore tube is to be used, such as a 32 to 34 French Gauge, without trocar and cannula, the following method may be employed. A number of holes are first cut in the side of the tube to improve drainage. The skin and muscle over the area are incised and the tube, held by a pair of forceps, is pushed upwards into the pleural cavity. The tube is then gently advanced for 7.5 to 10 cm and connected to the water-seal drainage system. The tube is then stitched in place or fixed to the skin as shown (Figure 36).

13. LUMBAR PUNCTURE

This procedure may be required in surgical wards as a diagnostic or therapeutic aid. It should not be performed if there is evidence of raised intracranial pressure. Since the spinal cord and meninges are involved, strict asepsis must be observed. A spinal needle, manometer and sterile containers for collecting cerebrospinal fluid (CSF) are required.

The patient is placed either on his side or sitting up. If on his side, he must be positioned at the very edge of the bed in the knee-chest position. This opens up the intervertebral space making the puncture easier. The operator, having scrubbed, and with mask and gloves on, prepares the area with antiseptic solution, if necessary after shaving the region. The puncture should be performed between the 3rd and 4th lumbar vertebrae. This space lies on a line joining the posterior superior iliac spines. Remember that in children the cord lies lower than this and may be injured at this level. It is best to use the space between L4 and L5 (Figure 37).

The region is infiltrated with local anaesthetic, making sure that the anaesthetic agent is infiltrated in the mid-line, which is relatively avascular. During the infiltration make sure that the needle is not at any time inserted to its full extent since sudden movement by the patient may cause it to snap, with subsequent difficulty in its removal.

While the local anaesthetic is acting check the equipment. Make sure that the needle and stilette fit and can be easily removed, and check that the manometer fits the attachment to the spinal needle. Have sterile containers ready if required. With everything set up the needle is then inserted through the same puncture mark. While pushing inwards with the right hand, the needle is steadied with the left. It is inserted in a slightly cranial direction for 4 to 5 cm. At this point, depending on the skin thickness of the individual, slight resistance will be felt. When this has been overcome the subarachnoid space will have been entered. The stilette is removed and clear cerebrospinal fluid should drip out.

The manometer is connected and the pressure measured

STERNAL MARROW PUNCTURE

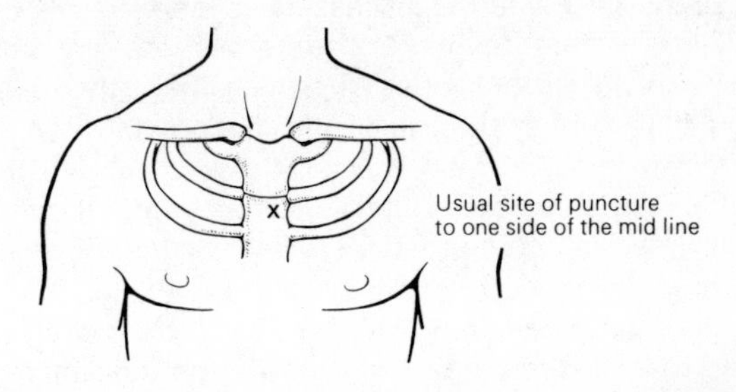

STERNAL MARROW PUNCTURE NEEDLE

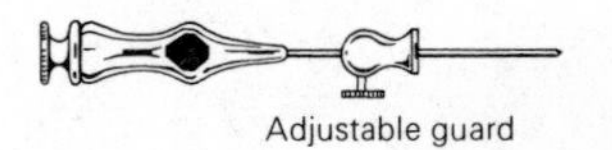

SITE OF LUMBAR PUNCTURE

Between 3rd and 4th lumbar vertebrae

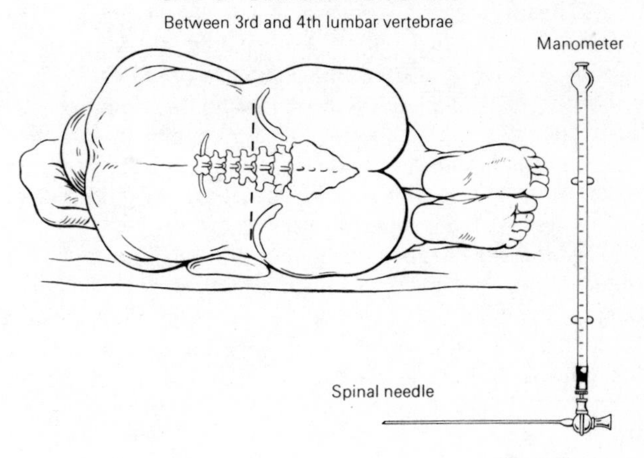

Figure 37

in centimetres of cerebrospinal fluid. If the subarachnoid space has no obstruction then the level of fluid in the manometer will move with respiration and the arterial pulse. To check free communication however the Queckenstedt test is applied. Momentary pressure is applied over both jugular veins. If communication is free then there should be a rise of 10 to 30 cm of water. After measuring the pressure a finger is placed over the top of the manometer tube which is then removed with the finger still over the tube; the column of CSF is placed over a sterile container and the finger removed. In this way precious CSF is not wasted. Further CSF is then removed if required by allowing it to drip from the needle. Finally the needle is withdrawn and the puncture hole sealed with a plastic spray and a light dressing applied. At the end of the procedure the patient remains in bed for a few hours, the foot of which is elevated.

The difficult lumbar puncture

1. **The restless patient.** This is particularly the case with children and confused adults. Careful handling and gentle restraint will usually allow the puncture to proceed normally.

2. **The dry tap.** If it is thought that the needle is in the subarachnoid space, then the needle should be rotated slightly in case it is pressing against a nerve root. If bone is encountered, it is likely that the needle has been inserted too vertically and it should be withdrawn and re-inserted in a more cranial direction. If no fluid is obtained by this manoeuvre the needle should be withdrawn completely and re-inserted in the space between L2 and L3.

3. **The bloody tap.** If this occurs it is important to try to differentiate between true blood in the CSF and contamination during the procedure. If contamination has been accidental then the blood will slowly decrease in volume and the fluid will become clear. If the CSF is truly blood-stained then the red colour will remain at the same intensity and when the red corpuscles have settled, the fluid will be yellow.

14. STERNAL MARROW PUNCTURE

Before starting this procedure it is worthwhile contacting the haematologist since he may wish to carry out the procedure himself, or prepare the slides. He will also be able to give advice as to the fixative to be used and supply any special containers required. A detailed explanation of the procedure is then given to the patient. Have ready local anaesthetic, the sternal marrow needle, a 20 ml syringe and watch glass to take the specimen of bone marrow. Preliminary pre-medication of the patient may be advisable (*see* Chapter 2).

After cleansing the skin over the sternum the area is towelled and the skin is anaesthetised down to the level of the periosteum. The most commonly used site is opposite the 2nd intercostal space, on one side of the midline (Figure 37). The periosteum must be properly anaesthetised if the procedure is to be performed painlessly. At this stage an estimate of the depth of the sternum is made and the guard of the sternal marrow needle adjusted accordingly. When anaesthesia is completed the needle is introduced using a gentle rotatory movement until the periosteum is reached. This is then penetrated by applying gentle, even pressure. The patient should be warned at this stage that a feeling of pressure may be experienced. The stilette is then removed, the syringe attached and suction applied. At this point the patient may experience a peculiar feeling of suction which may be distressing. Fears should be allayed by reassurance or better still by anticipation of the sensation.

In most cases bone marrow can be aspirated from this site though if the marrow is very hypoplastic, none may be obtained. If a 'dry tap' occurs another area of the sternum should be anaesthetised and the procedure repeated, usually at the level of a lower intercostal space. If no marrow can be obtained then the procedure should be abandoned and an iliac crest marrow puncture carried out.

When the marrow has been obtained it is rapidly placed in a watch glass containing citrate solution and small pieces of marrow picked up with a needle, placed on a slide, and a smear made using a second glass slide. A number of such slides are made. The remainder of the marrow is placed in fixative for further investigations. If not fixed immediately the slides should be taken to the haematology department forthwith.

While this is being carried out the stilette is replaced in the needle and the patient's attention held by an assistant or nurse so that he is not aware of the instrument which may appear to be penetrating his chest wall. When the slides have been prepared the stilette and needle are withdrawn and a dry dressing applied.

15. PREPARATION FOR RADIOLOGY

In this section emphasis is placed on the preparation of the patient for radiological procedures and on the principles of the techniques described. Although the houseman may be fully aware of the indications for radiology he may not know how to prepare his patients for them. The houseman should also be able to explain the nature of the procedure to be carried out so that the patient will appreciate the significance of the X-ray and be aware beforehand of the methods and instruments to be used. It goes without saying that full clinical information on the patient should be sent to the Radiology Department with the request for the examination.

Orthopaedic conditions

Little preparation of the patient is required. All clothing or radio-opaque material carried by the patient should be removed prior to X-ray. If a foreign body is suspected in the soft tissues of the body a marker is placed on the skin and two views of the area taken to facilitate subsequent exploration.

If a fracture is suspected at least two views of the bone are required. If necessary, the normal side is X-rayed for comparison. This is especially the case in children where developing epiphyses may cause some difficulty. Similarly if a dislocation is suspected two views are mandatory.

Chest X-ray

This is one of the most commonly carried out investigations and for it no preparation is required. Usually, a postero-anterior film is taken, but if the examination is carried out in the ward with a mobile machine then an antero-posterior view is obtained. The film is taken on full inspiration to show the maximum area of lung. For accurate localisation of fluid or masses within the thorax a lateral view is essential and tomography may be indicated. If a subphrenic abscess is suspected then screening of the diaphragm should be undertaken to detect limitation of movement. If a pneumothorax is thought to be present, films in both inspiration and expiration should be taken since a small pneumothorax may be visible only on expiration.

Angiography

Radiological examination of veins and arteries may be carried out under local or general anaesthesia. In most cases however the patient should be fasted and prepared for a general anaesthetic (Chapter 2). Premedication is essential in either case (Chapter 2).

1. **Angiocardiography.** Either local or general anaesthesia may be used. The right heart is catheterised by inserting a catheter from the ante-cubital or femoral veins under fluoroscopic control into the appropriate chamber. Left heart catheterisation is carried out using the femoral artery. The catheter is inserted by the Seldinger Method (*see* below) and is passed under fluoroscopic control. Alternatively for left heart catheterisation the right heart catheter may be used to pierce the interventricular septum.

2. **Arteriography.** Two methods are available. The first is direct arterial puncture and can be used for peripheral arteries, the carotids and vertebrals, and the abdominal aorta. The second involves percutaneous arterial catheterisation (Seldinger technique). A needle is inserted into the artery and through this a guide wire is passed. The needle is withdrawn and a catheter threaded over the guide wire into the artery. The femoral artery and axillary artery are the usual sites for this procedure. This method can be further refined in that various arteries, such as the renals, superior and inferior mesenteric and coeliac arteries may be selectively catheterised. For these investigations local or general anaesthesia may be used.

3. **Phlebography.** Several methods are available for the demonstration of veins of the lower and upper limbs, the venae cavae, the renal and adrenal veins. For the demonstration of veins of the lower limb a needle is inserted into a superficial vein over the dorsum of the foot and, by compression of the superficial veins, contrast medium is directed into the deep veins of the calf and thigh. This method may be

used to detect deep venous thrombosis or incompetent perforating veins.

A further method for the demonstration of the deep veins of the lower limb is the use of interosseous phlebography. General anaesthesia is used. A bone marrow needle is inserted through the cortex of the bone into the marrow and contrast medium injected. For the lower limb the needle may be placed in the calcaneum or in the medial or lateral malleoli. For demonstration of the ilio-femoral venous segments, pelvic veins and lower inferior vena cava, the contrast medium is injected into the greater trochanter of the femur.

For demonstration of the inferior vena cava, or selective venography of the renal veins, retrograde catheterisation via the femoral vein by the Seldinger technique may be used. These techniques can be performed under local anaesthesia.

Radiology of the portal system

This is most conveniently performed by percutaneous splenic puncture, under local anaesthesia. The spleen is punctured by a needle inserted through the 10th or 11th intercostal spaces in the mid-axillary line, the needle being passed inwards and upwards. When the capsule of the spleen has been entered, blood tracks back down the needle, especially if the portal pressure is raised. 20 to 50 ml of contrast medium are injected and a rapid series of films taken. Dye is carried via the splenic vein to the portal vein which, if patent, is outlined.

The portal vein may also be visualised by cannulating a radical of the superior mesenteric vein at operation. Recently the umbilical vein has been used for portal venous radiology A small upper mid-line abdominal incision is made and the vein identified extra-peritoneally. This is dilated then contrast medium is injected.

Lymphangiography

This may be used as a diagnostic procedure or as a therapeutic method for the insertion of cytotoxic agents into the lymphatics or lymph nodes. In most cases the lymphatics of the lower limbs and abdominal region are required to be visualised. The patient should be admitted for this procedure for two reasons. Firstly, late films at 24 and 48 hours are required. Secondly, close observation of the patient is required since pulmonary oil emboli may occur. The procedure is therefore contraindicated in patients with severe cardio-respiratory disease. Patients with iodine sensitivity, or with inter-digital infection should not have this examination.

If the leg is oedematous it should be elevated for 48 hours before the procedure. About one hour before the start of the investigation, 0.5 ml of patent blue violet is injected into the toe webs on the affected side. Over the next hour the superficial skin lymphatics will become visible and easy to identify. The patient's skin however, will also become blue or green for the following 24 to 48 hours and this should be explained to him at least the day before the procedure, so that relatives and visitors may be warned. During this period the urine is also blue or green.

An incision is then made on the dorsum of the foot and a lymphatic vessel identified and cannulated using a special needle and cannula. The contrast medium is injected slowly at a rate of 0.1 ml/minute using a pump. Films are taken of the legs, abdomen, pelvis and chest. An IVP is usually performed at the same time when a retroperitoneal glandular mass is suspected. At the end of the procedure the needle is removed and the wound closed.

Radiology of the gastrointestinal tract and abdomen

1. **The salivary glands.** Plain films of the salivary glands, parotid, submaxillary and sublingual using special views may show radio-opaque salivary calculi. More information may be obtained by sialography in which, after preliminary dilatation of the ducts, a fine catheter is introduced and 1 to 2 ml of viscous contrast medium injected. No anaesthesia is required.

2. **Pharynx and oesophagus.** A lateral soft tissue X-ray of the pharynx will give information about foreign bodies and bony damage in the area. A barium swallow however gives

fuller information. The X-rays are taken in the erect, supine and Trendelenburg, or head down, positions and the bolus of barium screened as it passes downwards. For a barium swallow the patient is prepared as for a barium meal since any pathology detected at the lower end of the oesophagus may necessitate this examination in addition.

3. **Stomach and duodenum.** These organs are visualised by the use of barium sulphate given as a barium meal. The patient is fasted for 12 hours prior to the examination. If pyloric stenosis is present, the stomach is washed out and nasogastric suction applied for a few days prior to the examination.

A barium sulphate/water mixture, 250 to 300 ml, is drunk. The first two mouthfuls are used as a barium swallow. The remainder is then swallowed and the stomach filled. Views are taken in oblique positions for visualisation of the stomach and duodenal cap. The patient is also viewed in the Trendelenburg position to examine for hiatus hernia and oesophageal regurgitation.

Radiological examination of the stomach in a patient with a haematemesis or melena stool is carried out as gently as possible using a small amount of barium sulphate or a water soluble medium such as 'Gastrografin'. By gentle rotation of the patient, adequate views can usually be obtained. If a nasogastric tube is in position, this may be used to instil the barium sulphate, and will also remove any blood or gastric juice which might obscure the picture.

Hypotonic duodenography using a mixture of barium sulphate and air, together with propantheline bromide ('Probanthine') is useful for visualising the duodenal loop.

4. **The small bowel.** Contrast medium is necessary for visualisation of the mucosal pattern of the small bowel. Several methods can be used. After a barium meal examination the barium may be followed through the small bowel. This has the disadvantage of depending on the rate of emptying of the stomach and this is not a continuous process. The normal barium sulphate mixture is not altogether suitable for outlining the small bowel since flocculation may occur. Accordingly a non-flocculating barium salt should be used.

Recently, neostigmine (0·5 mg i.v.) or metoclopramide ('Maxolon', 10 mg i.v.) have been used to give rapid emptying of the stomach with better visualisation of the small bowel. Alternatively a small bowel enema can be performed. A fine tube is passed orally into the third part of the duodenum and through this 20 to 30 ml of a non-flocculating barium salt is given. This is followed by 600 to 1200 ml of water which drives the barium to the ileocaecal valve outlining the whole small bowel. The patient should be warned that this examination may take up to five hours to complete.

5. **The colon.** Although some detail may be visible in the straight X-ray of abdomen, a barium enema is the most usual radiological investigation. Preliminary preparation of the patient with an enema is essential to clear out faeces and give a good view of the mucosa. A rectal tube is inserted into the patient and barium allowed to run in, by gravity, under fluoroscopic control. Films are taken of special areas and lateral X-rays of the pelvi-rectal junction taken for detailed visualisation of this region.

A double contrast enema is carried out by radiological examination after partial defaecation of the barium. This may take some time and evacuation may be hastened by the introduction of air into the colon to displace the barium. This part of the procedure may be unpleasant to the patient.

6. **Plain X-rays of the abdomen.** Plain X-rays of the abdomen may be useful for diagnostic purposes particularly in the acute abdomen. It is important that good films are obtained and that both erect and supine films, and films to show the diaphragms are taken. The erect and supine films will show whether or not fluid levels are present in the gastrointestinal tract. If the patient is too ill to be examined in the erect position, a lateral decubitus view with the patient on his side will be helpful and less disturbing to the patient. Views of the diaphragms in the erect position are essential if the patient is suspected of having a perforated viscus.

Sinograms

In patients with a persistently discharging sinus of the abdominal wall, or any other area, often related to previous surgery, the instillation of dye into the sinus will give information as to its cause and relation to underlying bowel or other viscus.

The biliary tract.

A plain X-ray taken without preparation of the patient may show the presence of gallstones in the gallbladder or bile ducts. Air in the biliary tract may be demonstrated by this method.

Oral cholecystography is the most common investigation. A plain film is taken the day before the examination. Twelve hours before the X-ray is to be performed the patient is given a preparation of an oral contrast medium such as 'Biloptin'. Very often the gallbladder and bile ducts are visualised by this method alone. A fatty meal or a commercial preparation such as Sorbital is then given to make the gallbladder contract. This makes visualisation of the bile ducts easier. In the presence of obstructive jaundice however, when the bilirubin level is greater than 4 mg per cent, the oral cholecystogram is of little use.

The four day Telepaque test may render non-opaque stones opaque. Telepaque 3 g is given orally over four days after which the usual views of the gallbladder area are taken. The contrast medium, given over this period of time, coats the stones making them identifiable.

Intravenous cholangiography

Using an intravenously given dye, concentrated by the liver, the hepatic and bile ducts can be readily visualised. It is particularly useful where detailed examination of the common bile duct is required or where the gallbladder has not been outlined by oral cholecystography. To carry out the test the dye is given intravenously and appears in the common bile duct in 15 to 20 minutes. Films are then taken for up to two hours, tomography being carried out at the same time if required. Once again, if the bilirubin level is greater than 4 mg per cent, little useful information will be gained.

Radiology of the common bile duct

The common bile duct may be outlined radiologically other than by oral or intravenous cholangiography. Operative cholangiography is carried out while the patient is in the operating theatre with the common bile duct exposed. A needle is inserted into the common bile duct, or into the cystic duct if cholecystectomy has been performed, and dye injected. This outlines the common bile duct and hepatic ducts and shows up obstruction in the ducts or the presence of stones. It is usually necessary to contact the radiologist the day before the operation to arrange the timing of the procedure.

In the post-operative period radiology of the common bile duct may be carried out using the T-tube which has been inserted into the duct at the time of operation. Before removal of the tube an X-ray should be carried out to ensure that there is no evidence of obstruction.

In the presence of obstructive jaundice, oral and intravenous cholecystography are of little use. In this situation, if information is required on the calibre and patency of the bile ducts, percutaneous transhepatic cholangiography may be considered. Under local anaesthesia a needle is passed into the liver and by manipulation placed into a dilated bile duct. Contrast medium is then injected and the biliary tree outlined. This investigation should be used only as a preliminary to operation. With this procedure, there is a high incidence of biliary leakage which will require operative treatment. Before the procedure, the patient should be prepared for theatre, blood should be available, and a course of vitamin K given. Infusion cholangiography may also be employed in this situation. The patient is given an intravenous infusion of contrast medium over a period of one hour, after which tomography is carried out.

Radiology of the urinary tract

The most common radiological examination of the urinary tract is the intravenous pyelogram (IVP). Preliminary preparation is necessary if good films are to be obtained. The bowel should be cleared by giving purgatives for the two days prior to radiology. With the conventional low dose IVP where 20 ml of the contrast medium is given, preliminary dehydration is necessary. The patient is allowed only 600 ml of fluid in the 24 hours before the X-ray, and none in the 12 hours prior to the procedure. If an IVP is required as an emergency where dehydration is not possible, a high dosage IVP is performed. A control film is taken, then a small dose of contrast medium (2 to 5 ml) is given intravenously to test for a reaction to iodine. If an adverse reaction occurs, Phenergan 20 to 50 mg is given intravenously followed by 100 mg of hydrocortisone. If no reaction occurs then 50 ml of the contrast solution ('urografin' 60, 'hypaque' 45 per cent) is given and films taken at 5 minutes and 20 minutes. This is usually sufficient to give the information required. Where a high dose IVP is performed preliminary dehydration is still considered desirable.

If for any reason, such as renal failure, an IVP fails to give an adequate view of the kidneys and ureters then cystoscopy followed by retrograde pyelography is carried out. A fine catheter is passed up each ureter in turn and dilute contrast medium injected. The cystoscopy may be performed under local or general anaesthesia and the patient should be prepared accordingly. Alternatively infusion pyelography with tomography may be useful.

Micturating cystography

The patient is first asked to empty the bladder and a urethral catheter is passed with full aseptic precautions. The bladder is filled with contrast medium and films taken. The patient is asked to micturate and a rapid series of films taken to show reflux of contrast medium into the ureters.

Injection urethrography in the male

This investigation is indicated in urethral injuries or urethral stricture. It should not be carried out in the presence of urethritis or balanitis. After emptying the bladder a viscous contrast medium is injected and films are taken in various positions.

Ultrasonic examination

This technique is useful in distinguishing solid from cystic masses. It is particularly useful in renal or retroperitoneal lesions, pancreatic cysts or aneurysms. It has of course a special place in the diagnosis of pelvic masses, ovarian or intra-uterine. No preparation of the patient is required, though the presence of a full bladder is of assistance.

16. THE MANAGEMENT OF CARDIAC ARREST

There is little use in knowing how to manage a cardiac arrest if the relevant apparatus and equipment are not available or cannot be located easily. The first essential therefore is to check the Ward or Recovery Room for the exact location of the laryngoscope and endotracheal tubes, ventilation bag with proper connections, the electrocardiogram machine, the portable defibrillator with electrical plugs and adaptors if necessary, and a suction machine. In addition sodium bicarbonate (8.4 per cent solution) together with other drugs, needles and syringes of various sizes, and equipment for intravenous infusions should be available. It is therefore convenient to have a 'cardiac arrest' trolley or tray available, situated in a strategic place in the Ward or Recovery Room. This must be regularly checked and drugs and equipment renewed as required. Many hospitals have a cardiac arrest team which can be available within a few minutes. Make sure you know how to call this team. Speed is of the utmost importance, so it is worthwhile rehearsing the cardiac arrest drill with the nursing staff since they will usually be first on the scene.

Cardiac arrest drill

The priorities are:

1. Adequate ventilation of the patient must be ensured immediately.

2. External cardiac massage should be commenced.

3. The cardiac arrest team or further assistance should be summoned.

The patient should be placed immediately on a firm surface, such as the floor or, if available, a special board placed under the mattress. The time should be noted. Although two persons are usually required the initial management can be carried out by one person while help is being summoned.

EXPIRED AIR RESUSCITATION

Mouth-to-mouth resuscitation tube

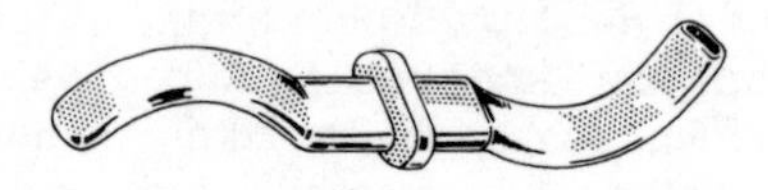

METHOD OF MOUTH-TO-MOUTH RESPIRATION FOR EXPIRED AIR RESUSCITATION

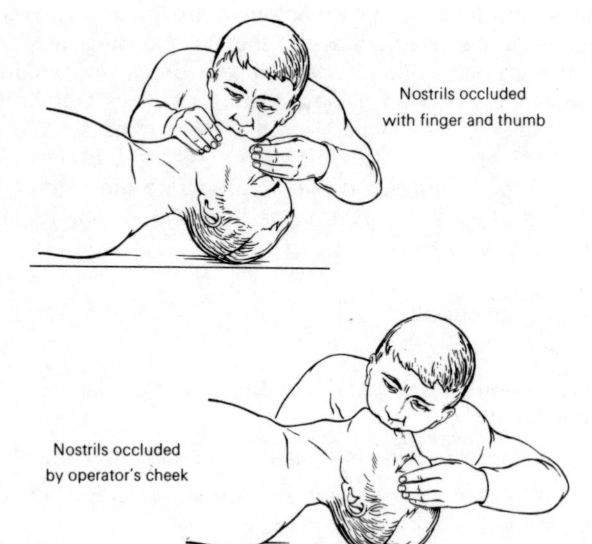

Figure 38

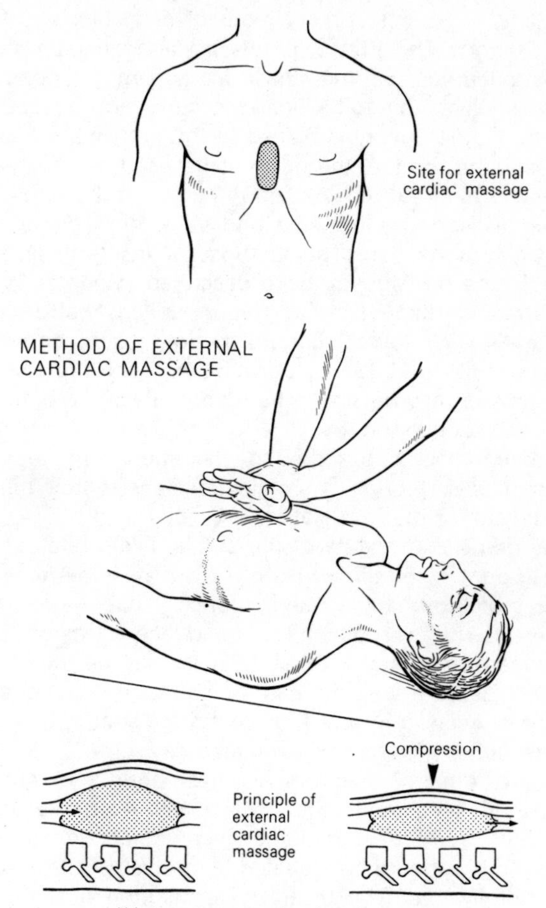
EXTERNAL CARDIAC MASSAGE
Site for external cardiac massage
METHOD OF EXTERNAL CARDIAC MASSAGE
Compression
Principle of external cardiac massage
Heart compressed against thoracic vertebrae

Figure 39

Ventilation may initially be carried out using the expired air method (mouth-to-mouth respiration) (Figure 38). With the operator on the right side of the patient the jaw is pulled forwards and upwards, the nose compressed with the left hand, and by direct contact expired air is blown into the patient's lungs. The efficacy of this procedure can be checked by the adequacy of the chest movement. A number of airways are available to facilitate mouth to mouth respiration. One end of the airway is placed in the patient's mouth and depresses the tongue, the other being used by the operator to deliver expired air. An endotracheal tube should be inserted as soon as possible and ventilation begun using 100 per cent oxygen. The method for inserting an endotracheal tube has already been described (Chapter 11).

External cardiac massage (Figure 39) is performed by compressing the lower sternum forcibly, using both hands at a rate of 60 to 100 beats per minute. Since the volume of blood moved may be small, the higher rate is the better. The sternum is depressed by 2 to 5 cm. The efficacy of the procedure may be checked by the palpation of the femoral or carotid pulses, though it should be realised that this may indicate transmitted pulsation not blood flow. A better clinical guide is the state of the pupils. Fixed dilated pupils indicate poor cerebral perfusion. Excessive force may cause fractures of the ribs and haemothorax or haemopericardium may result. The heart may be torn and lacerations of the liver and spleen may occur. This however, may be inevitable in elderly patients if external cardiac massage is adequate. At the end of every fourth or fifth beat there should be a pause and the patient should be ventilated.

Once external cardiac massage has begun and ventilation established, an intravenous infusion should be set up and 100 mEq of sodium bicarbonate given immediately to correct acidosis. This should be repeated at intervals if the resuscitation is prolonged. The bicarbonate solution may be given through an intravenous giving set or directly into the femoral vein. A cut-down may be required. If resuscitation is successful arterial blood should be taken and the acid-base status of the patient assessed and corrected as required.

An electrocardiograph should be obtained as soon as possible to determine the next therapeutic measure. If ventricular fibrillation is present then the heart should be defibrillated. Both A.C. and D.C. machines are available. With a portable A.C. defibrillator machine, one electrode is placed over the left sternal edge and the other over the anterior axillary line. All personnel should be out of contact with the patient before defibrillation is attempted. A single shock of 250 volts is given and this may be repeated up to five times, the voltage being increased to 750 volts. Direct current defibrillation is more effective but requires more elaborate apparatus which may be part of the cardiac arrest equipment. If defibrillation is unsuccessful internal cardiac massage with direct cardiac defibrillation may be attempted. Should the defibrillation be reversed and the patient reverts to a sinus rhythm, an intravenous infusion of lignocaine (1 to 2 mg/kg in 5 per cent dextrose) should be commenced after a loading dose of 1 to 2 mg/kg.

If asystole is present, a sharp blow to the chest may restart the heart. If this is unsuccessful, intracardiac adrenaline (5 ml of 1:10,000 solution) given by direct intracardiac puncture may be of value. Alternatively 5 ml of 10 per cent calcium chloride may be given, again by the intracardiac route. It should be recognised that these drugs may act because of the direct mechanical stimulation of the heart by the needle during administration. If these methods are unsuccessful then external cardiac pacing or internal cardiac massage may be required. If the electrocardiograph shows a weak but spontaneous heart beat, pressor agents such as isoprenaline, 0·1 mg, should be given intravenously, and repeated according to the clinical state of the patient. External cardiac massage should be continued during this time.

Internal cardiac massage

This method is more efficient than external cardiac massage and is less tiring if resuscitation is to be continued for some time. It is usually restricted to patients with asystole for whom it has been decided that resuscitation should be continued for some time.

A long incision from the left sternal border to the posterior axillary line in the 4th or 5th intercostal spaces is made. After incising the skin the intercostal muscle and parietal pleura are then divided, care being taken not to damage the underlying lung or heart. The ribs are then retracted and the right hand inserted, the heart being massaged against the sternum at a rate of 60 beats per minute. If this does not result in spontaneous heart beat then the pericardium should be incised and both hands inserted and the heart massaged. Intracardiac adrenaline, calcium or isoprenaline may then be given.

Post-resuscitation care

This is a specialised area of patient care since the patient will require intensive and continuous monitoring for some time after the incident.

COMPLICATIONS

Although CVP measurements are of enormous help in situations of hypovolaemia and to a lesser extent myocardial infarction, venous catheters may be associated with complications and they should not therefore be used unless a definite therapeutic advantage is expected. The following complications have all been recorded.

(1) Thrombophlebitis. This is almost inevitable if the catheter is left in for more than 10 days and is probably due to mechanical irritation. The inflammation is rapidly settled by short-wave therapy but a blocked vein is inevitable and occasionally oedema of the upper arm results.
(2) Infection of the cut-down site[4]. This is minimised by scrupulous aseptic technique and polybactrine spray. It is also a good idea to separate the sites of entry of the catheter through the skin and into the vein as far as possible.
(3) Infection of the catheter tip is less easily avoided and may give rise to septicaemia. At any rate, it is a wise precaution to culture the catheter tip after it has been removed.
(4) Erosion of the vein. If this is not recognised early it may cause widespread infusion of fluid into subcutaneous tissues, which is painful for the patient and may be dangerous if secondary infection occurs. If suspected, the catheter should be withdrawn.
(5) Arterial bleeding sufficient to cause tracheal obstruction is a potential complication of all jugular and subclavian puncture techniques.
(6) Pneumothorax is a specific complication of subclavian vein puncture.
(7) Catheter embolus into the right heart is known to occur if the catheter is inadvertently broken at the site of entry to the skin. Surgical advice should be sought.

THE SWAN-GANZ CATHETER[3]

Pulmonary wedge pressure

Knowledge of the left and right atrial pressures is essential for the informed management of complicated acute heart failure. It is also wise to have an arterial cannula for continuous monitoring of pressure and for blood gas analysis. Finally, cardiac output measurement, perhaps something of a luxury, provides all the information necessary to manage the most complex haemodynamic problems.

The Swan-Ganz catheter

Right atrial pressure is measured with a CVP line (*see* p. 239), whilst left atrial pressure is most conveniently measured using a flow directed pulmonary artery catheter (Swan-Ganz catheter). This can be put in at the bedside without X-ray control. The left atrial pressure at which pulmonary oedema will appear is dependent on the serum albumin. A simple formula expresses this dependence (*see* p. 30).

(A) **The catheter**

Has two lumens, one of which controls a balloon immediately behind the catheter tip, whilst the other opens as a single end-hole. The balloon has a dual function; during insertion it is blown-up (with air or CO_2) as soon as the catheter tip is in a central vein. Thereafter the balloon acts as a sail, directing the catheter tip in the direction of maximal flow i.e. through the tricuspid and pulmonary valves. Once the tip is in a small pulmonary artery, inflation of the balloon will occlude the artery proximally, leaving the end-hole exposed to the pulmonary capillary pressure (pulmonary wedge pressure), which is assumed to be identical with left atrial pressure.

Swan-Ganz catheters are usually available in two sizes:

7F with a 1·5cc balloon
5F with a 0·8cc balloon

We have found the larger size easier to manipulate and less likely to clot. For cardiac output measurement, using the thermodilution technique, catheters are available with an additional injection lumen in the right atrium and two thermistors beyond.

(B) *Catheter insertion* is best by an antecubital cutdown on the basilic vein – a technique free of serious complications. Alternatively the